Delivering Quality in Midwifery

CC
D

Delivering Quality in Midwifery

E. Rosemary Buckley

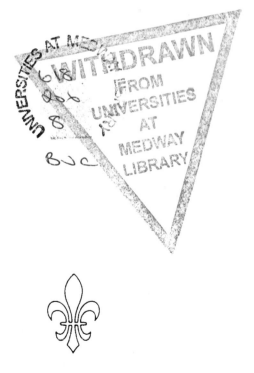

Baillière Tindall
London Philadelphia Toronto Sydney Tokyo

Baillière Tindall   24–28 Oval Road
London NW1 7DX

The Curtis Center
Independence Square West
Philadelpia, PA 19106-3399, USA

Harcourt Brace & Company
55 Horner Avenue
Toronto, Ontario, M8Z 4X6, Canada

Harcourt Brace & Company, Australia
30–52 Smidmore Street
Marrickville
NSW 2204, Australia

Harcourt Brace & Company, Japan
Ichibancho Central Building
22–1 Ichibancho
Chiyoda-ku, Tokyo 102, Japan

A catalogue record for this book is available from the British Library

ISBN 0–7020–2134–2

Typeset by Saxon Graphics Ltd, Derby
Printed and bound in Great Britain by
WBC, Bridgend, Mid Glamorgan

Contents

Foreword

Midwives should welcome this first book on the delivery of quality care in midwifery. It has been written by Rosemary Buckley, a practising midwife. The author has been involved in clinical audit and quality of midwifery care for several years, and this book is the culmination of her wide experience gained following her appointment as senior midwife to carry out skill mix and dependancy studies and subsequently as quality assurance coordinator in a busy maternity unit.

The book has a well researched base and shows clearly the need for audit and quality in the midwifery profession. It fills a gap in our current knowledge and practice.

It will help midwives at grass roots to become more confident at measuring the effectiveness of the care they give, safe in the knowledge that it is based on expertise that has been gained by a colleague while working in the field.

Attention should be paid to Section 4 which provides an excellent description of the management of change and is worthy of particular study.

Midwives will find the examples contained in the book to be topical and relevant to their everyday practice. Managers will discover that the value of setting up a system of quality assurance as described will far outweigh the resources required to give the optimum amount of care to the mothers and babies in the maternity services, as well as increased job satisfaction and the raising of staff morale.

Margaret B. McIntosh

Ackowledgements

This book would not have been possible without the original vision of Mrs Margaret McIntosh (Senior Midwifery Manager, now retired) in 1991 to implement quality assurance in the Nottingham City Hospital Maternity Unit.

Neither would this book have been possible without the ideas, involvement and work of midwifery, medical, auxilliary and clerical staff at the Nottingham City Hospital Maternity Unit, especially members of the Antenatal Clinic, Wards and Labour Suite Standard Setting Groups. My ackowledgements and thanks go to all of them.

Ackowledgements and thanks particularly go to Gill Bradley, Lorraine Hargreaves, Jackie Parkin, Robert Dawson and Ben Halliday for help and support with quality initiatives, and to May Cox-Brown (Senior Midwifery Manager) for permission to publish results from audits carried out in the Maternity Unit.

Lastly, special thanks are due to Val Ranyard and Michyla Hickling for their very patient proof-reading, help and advice with this book, and to all friends, family, colleagues and the staff at Baillière Tindall who have helped and encouraged me in this venture.

Rosemary Buckley

Section *1* Introducing Quality

1 Why Quality?

Quality is not a new idea. It has been around since the
beginning of the world when 'God saw all that He had
made, and it was very good' (*Genesis* ch.1 v.31). People too
have always been able to judge quality for themselves.

A short history of quality and audit in the health care professions

The history of quality in the health care professions goes
back a long way. The earliest record of standards in health
care are from Greek and Roman times, one of which is the
Hippocratic oath (Ellis and Whittington, 1993).

In 1518, the Royal College of Physicians produced a charter 'to uphold the standards of practice both for their own honour and for public benefit' (Ellis and Whittington, 1993). However, it is Florence Nightingale who is recognized as probably one of the first health professionals to actually evaluate health care and implement change as a result (Crombie *et al.*, 1993; Maxwell, 1984; Walshe and Coles, 1993; Ellis and Whittington, 1993; Sale, 1991; Marr and Giebing, 1994). During the Crimean War she showed that deaths in hospital were more likely to be due to hospital-acquired infections than injuries sustained on the battle field and introduced standards of care that drastically reduced the mortality rate from infection (Maxwell, 1984). Within six months of her arrival at the hospital at Scutari, Turkey, mortality rates had fallen from 40% to 2% (Crombie *et al.* 1993).

Subsequently, on her return to Britain, Florence Nightingale investigated hospital mortality rates and considered how they could be improved. She placed great emphasis on accurate and systematic collection and evaluation of hospital statistics so that comparisons could be made between different wards. On comparing mortality rates between hospitals she found large differences between them and concluded that 'facts such as these have sometimes raised grave doubts as to the advantages to be derived from hospitals at all, and have led one to think that in all probability a poor sufferer would have a much better chance of recovery if treated at home'! (Nightingale, 1863). She went on to set standards and implement change as a result of her findings.

Nightingale's work on surgical mortality was developed by a surgeon, E.W. Groves, who attempted to compare surgical mortality between hospitals. He called for a standardized classification of operations and diseases and publication of surgical outcomes by a central authority to provide 'valuable knowledge as to the prognosis after operations' and other information (Groves, 1908; Walshe and Coles, 1993).

In the late nineteenth century midwives strove to become recognized as a profession and the Midwives Institute was established in 1881 to unite midwives and provide pressure for a Midwives Act, which eventually came into force in 1902. The aim of the organization was 'to encourage the training of midwives so as to lead to a better standard of care for mothers and babies,' a continued aim of the (now) Royal College of Midwives in the century since its foundation (Cowell and Wainwright, 1981).

Codman was an American surgeon at the beginning of the twentieth century who studied outcomes as a measure of success. He followed up his patients a year after operation, looking at outcomes such as accuracy of the original diagnosis, success of the operation and side effects (Codman, 1914; Maxwell, 1984; Ellis and Whittington, 1993; Walshe and Coles, 1993).

Isabel Stewart (1919) looked at ways of measuring the quality of nursing care and the effective use of resources, and in 1936 Carter and Balme published a book about evaluating care which recommended regular multidisciplinary review of all patients on the ward.

There was little subsequent interest in quality of health care in the UK, it flourished in the USA in the 1950s and 1960s. Indeed, Maxwell (1984), a British author, stated that 'Arguably, no conceptual advance has been made since Codman.'

One important initiative did, however, become established. *The Confidential Enquiry into Maternal Deaths* was instituted in 1952, and was the first nationwide clinical audit. It grew out of a series of similar enquiries in the 1920s and 1930s. The enquiry looks into maternal deaths occurring during pregnancy, labour and the puerperium. An investigation is carried out and the results collated into a triennial report. Recommendations are made based on the findings. The Enquiry has been credited with reducing maternal deaths since it was started (Maxwell, 1984; Department of Health, 1991a).

Other national audits have since been established including *The Confidential Enquiry into Stillbirths and Deaths in Infancy* (CESDI) introduced by the Department of Health in 1993. Details of all fetal and neonatal deaths from 20 weeks, gestation up to one year of age are collected and sent to central points in each region. An annual report is produced, making recommendations where appropriate.

A milestone in quality in health care was established when Avedis Donabedian published his paper laying the foundations of quality theory and outlining the basics of 'structure, process, outcome' (1966) which he later expanded in his book *The Definition of Quality and Approaches to its Assessment* (1980). Donabedian's model went on to become the most influential and widely used model in health care (Kitson, 1989; Walshe and Coles, 1993).

Maxwell (1984) proposed an alternative model in an article in the *British Medical Journal* that famously outlined the dimensions of quality. Health care organizations have used these dimensions to set and evaluate standards of health care.

Others have developed quality models, usually based on Donabedian's work, including Charles Shaw who wrote *Introducing Quality Assurance* in 1987 and CRM Wilson, whose work built on that of Donabedian and who wrote *Hospital-Wide Quality Assurance*, also in 1987. An influential person in the field of nursing is Professor Alison Kitson who was instrumental in developing the *Dynamic Standard Setting System (DySSSy)* and whose work is built on the earlier studies of Clark and Kendall, which in turn was based on the seminal work of Donabedian (Royal College of Nursing (RCN), 1990).

In 1985, Britain and other European member states signed a declaration that they would establish effective mechanisms for quality assurance in their health care systems by 1990 (World Health Organization, 1985).

In 1989 the Government released a white paper *Working for Patients* (Department of Health, 1989). This included a statement that 'local managers, in consultation with their professional colleagues, will be expected to re-examine all areas of work to identify the most cost-effective use of professional skills. This may involve a re-appraisal of traditional patterns and practices."

In response, Project 32 was set up to address how this aim might be implemented in the nursing and midwifery professions. The *Framework of Audit for Nursing Services* was produced as a result (Department of Health, 1991b). It defined nursing audit as an activity in which all nurses, midwives and health visitors should be involved, and suggested ways of implementing audit into all areas of nursing and midwifery: clinical, managerial and organizational.

The climate of audit and quality had therefore become established and professional organizations representing the different health disciplines (*Box 1.1*)

Box 1.1   *Professional bodies' quality and audit initiatives*

- 1965 The Royal College of Nursing

- 1975 The Royal College of Radiologists

- 1977 The Royal College of Physicians

- 1983 Royal College of General Practitioners

- 1987 Royal College of Surgeons

- 1989 Royal College of Occupational Therapists

- 1990 Chartered Society of Physiotherapists

- 1991 College of Speech and Language Therapists

started to produce standards or statements about quality and audit issues.

In 1995, a joint working group of the Royal College of Obstetricians and Gynaecologists and the Royal College of Midwives produced a report on communication standards with the aim among others 'to define the need for the provision of minimum standards of information for patients undergoing obstetric/midwifery procedures and to draw up appropriate standards of communication' (Royal College of Obstetricians and Gynaecologists, 1995).

It can be seen that over the centuries quality and audit issues have become an increasingly important and indeed a central part of practice in the health professions, particularly in clinical practice. Midwives themselves formalized their desire for good standards of care for mothers and babies as far back as 1881 and continue to do so to the present day.

Definitions of quality

Many terms are used to describe and discuss audit and quality. Shaw (1992) showed that terms associated with quality and audit could be combined to produce 96 phrases that either have been or could be used to mean review of health care. Shaw (1987) also stated that 'Watertight definitions of quality and related terms are too elusive to merit the time of practical people!' Nevertheless, it is often helpful to at least attempt to capture the meaning of the various terms (*Boxes 1.2–1.4*).

Box 1.2   Quality

- 'Degree of excellence' (*The Little Oxford Dictionary*, 1980)

- 'Quality is what you like' (Pirsig, 1974)

- 'Quality is conformance with requirements' (Crosby, 1979)

- 'That which satisfies the customer' (Ellis and Whittington, 1993)

- 'The definition of quality may be almost anything any-one wants it to be, although it is, ordinarily, a reflection of values and goals current in the medical care system and in the larger society of which it is a part' (Donabedian, 1966)

Box 1.3   Quality service

- 'A quality service ... gives people what they need as well as what they want at lowest cost' (Ovretveit, 1992)

- 'The application of all necessary services of modern medicine to the needs of all people' (Lee and Jones, 1933)

- 'The conformity between actual care and preset criteria' (Donabedian, 1970)

- 'The extent to which the care provided is expected to achieve the most favourable balance of risks and benefits' (Donabedian, 1980)

- 'Reviewing the quality of services and taking action to sustain what is good and improve on what is not' (King's Fund, 1986)

Box 1.4   Quality assurance

> ● 'Quality assurance is a management system by means of which we assure ourselves and others of the quality of work for which we have responsibility' (Wilson, 1987)
>
> ● 'Quality assurance is the measurement of the actual level of the service provided plus the efforts to modify, when necessary, the provision of these services in the light of the results of the measurement' (Williamson, 1978)

The term quality assurance is synonymous with quality improvement.

Definitions of audit

The word audit comes from the Latin word 'audire', which means 'to hear' and refers to oral reports of financial accounts. This original meaning is reflected in the dictionary definition of audit as an 'official examination of accounts' (*The Little Oxford Dictionary*, 1980). Other definitions are given in *Box 1.5*.

Audit or research?

Audit and research have similar functions. Both seek to increase knowledge, often by similar methods. There are differences though: research aims to be generalizable whereas audit is usually carried out at a local level and the

Box 1.5   Definitions of audit

- 'Official examination of accounts' (*The Little Oxford Dictionary*, 1980)

- 'Systematic measurement with a view to evaluation' (Buckley, unpublished)

- 'Audit focuses on the way care is delivered to identify reasons for inadequate care' (Crombie *et al.*, 1993)

- 'Clinical audit is the process by which medical staff collectively review, evaluate and improve their practice' (Frostick *et al.*, 1993)

- 'Nursing audit is part of the cycle of quality assurance. It incorporates the systematic and critical analyses by nurses, midwives and health visitors, in conjunction with other staff of the planning, delivery and evaluation of nursing and midwifery care, in terms of their use of resources and the outcomes for patients/clients, and introduces appropriate change in response to that analysis' (Department of Health, 1993)

---

findings relate to and apply at that level. Research often involves controlled trials, audit never does. Research is concerned with finding out what should happen, while audit is concerned with finding out what is actually happening. The quotes in *Box 1.6* show the differences in emphasis.

Box 1.6   Differences between audit and research

- 'Research is concerned with discovering the right thing to do: audit with ensuring it is done right' (Smith, 1992)

- 'Clinical research is undertaken when a prospective controlled trial is instituted. Audit of clinical care is the assessment of clinical care provided for an individual or group of patients. The audit is undertaken retrospectively (on hopefully, prospectively acquired data) and will examine the usual form of treatment that a particular clinician provides' (Frostick et al., 1993)

- 'Research is the scientific study to determine what constitutes good care and what should be done, i.e. standards of care. Audit is the scientific study of whether the standards are being met' (Maresh, 1994)

- '... randomised controlled trials and clinical audit can to some extent be seen as two ends of a single process involving dissemination, education and change management' (Firth-Cozens, 1996)

- 'Audit should be conducted with as much scientific rigour as clinical research projects' (Maresh, 1994)

Audit or quality?

The definitions of some words evolve with time. Audit appears to be one of them. The narrower and earlier definitions of audit confine it to measuring or examining with little relation to context. However, the term audit, as related to health care, seems to be evolving to adopt the same meaning as quality in that quality and audit cycles are often presented as almost identical concepts. For example 'Audit is the process used by health professionals to assess, evaluate and improve the care of patients in a systematic way in order to enhance their health and quality of life' (Irvine and Irvine, 1991). It appears that the concept of audit has broadened from the narrow definition of measurement, only to include evaluation and the steps taken to implement change as a result of that evaluation.

The constituents of quality

Maxwell (1984) outlined the dimensions of quality as access to services, relevance to need (for the whole community), effectiveness, equity, social acceptability, efficiency and economy. It might be added that a quality service should also be ethical (*Box 1.7*).

Box 1.7   A quality service should be ...

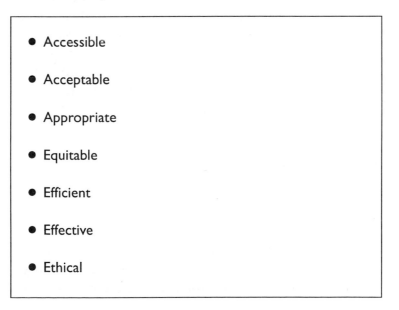

- Accessible

- Acceptable

- Appropriate

- Equitable

- Efficient

- Effective

- Ethical

Why quality in midwifery?

From biblical times, midwives have been concerned with providing high quality care to mothers and babies. They have not been so good, however, at evaluating the care that they give. There are several reasons why it is important that quality issues should be central to midwives' practice.

Professional and Statutory Accountability

Midwives' practice has been regulated by statute since the Midwives Act of 1902. The United Kingdom Central Council for Nursing, Midwifery and Health Visiting (1994) states that 'the exercise of accountability requires the practitioner to seek to achieve and maintain high standards.'

It was Auld in 1979 at a Royal College of Midwives conference, who first articulated the need for midwives to audit their practice and set standards of care (Auld, 1980). She said that the profession had, at that time 'not attempted to evaluate with any degree of accuracy or certainty the care given, nor have we established a code of good practice with a clarity that can be understood by all.' Her call went largely unheeded. An extensive search of the literature found little reference to quality initiatives in midwifery between 1975 and 1993 (Dawson, 1993). This situation is, however, starting to be rectified as midwives become more aware of the need to systematically examine, and evaluate practice and to implement change on the basis of their findings.

Government

In 1989, the Department of Health issued the white paper *Working for Patients*, which stated that 'local managers in consultation with their professional colleagues, will be expected to re-examine all areas of work to identify the most cost-effective use of professional skills. This may involve a re-appraisal of traditional patterns and practices' (Department of Health, 1989). In this way the government placed a requirement on all health professionals to review their practice.

In 1991, The Department of Health became more specific in relation to nurses, midwives and health visitors as follows: 'Nursing audit is part of the cycle of quality assurance. It incorporates the systematic and critical analyses by nurses, midwives and health visitors, in conjunction with other staff, of the planning, delivery and evaluation of nursing and midwifery care, in terms of their use of resources and the outcomes for patient/clients and introduces appropriate change in response to that analysis' (Department of Health, 1991a).

Working parallel to these initiatives was *The Patients Charter*, which stated as its aim to give 'a service which puts the patient first, providing services that meet clearly defined national and local standards' (Department of Health, 1991c).

In 1993 the document *Changing Childbirth* directed at maternity services was produced. It stated that 'there is a long history in maternity services of well-intentioned changes which are not backed-up with proper research-based evidence to support their introduction.' It went on to say 'clinical practice should be based on sound evidence and be subject to regular clinical audit' (Department of Health, 1993). The government has therefore placed a requirement and responsibility on midwives to base their practice on research and to systematically evaluate their practice to demonstrate that they are delivering a quality service.

Lay Bodies

Lay bodies such as the Association for the Improvement

in Maternity Services (AIMS) and National Childbirth Trust (NCT) represent the public to an extent and have put pressure on midwives to improve the service they provide. Midwives are accountable to the public for their practice.

Mothers

Mothers, of course, are the most important reason why midwives should give quality care. As the health professionals who have the major input into the care of mothers and babies, it is vital that the care midwives give is evaluated and, where necessary, improved.

In addition, since the advent of *The Patient's Charter* (Department of Health, 1991c), consumers of health services have become more aware of their rights and are much quicker to complain about shortcomings in the service or care they receive. Bark *et al.* (1994) state that complaints have increased fivefold. The recent publication of the complaints leaflet entitled *Complaints: Listening... Acting...Improving* by the NHS Executive (Department of Health, 1996) emphasizes the consumer's rights and putting an obligation on health care providers to respond to complaints. Maternity services are not immune. Bark *et al.* (1994) found that 8% of complaints involved maternity services. For many mothers maternity care will be their first experience of hospitals and health care staff, and expectations will be high at this important point in their lives. Mothers and their relatives are much quicker to complain now than in the past about waiting in clinics, poor staff attitudes, inadequate explanations and shortcomings in care. Mothers have a right to expect high standards of care. However, midwives are human like everyone else, and mistakes are made. Implementing quality into maternity services is an effective way of improving the service and demonstrating that staff are serious about providing high quality care.

Quality is not an Option

Why should midwives involve themselves in quality issues? There is not really an option. Professionally, midwives are accountable for their own practice and need to demonstrate that the care they give is 'good practice,' effective and research-based, and where there are no research findings that it is based on professionally agreed consensus standards.

Changing Childbirth (Department of Health, 1993) and other government papers require that midwives systematically evaluate and improve their practice. Lay bodies also want their say in how, maternity services are delivered. Lastly, and very importantly, midwives have a duty to provide the mothers and babies they care for the best possible service.

Quality methods

There are many different methods of introducing quality. Some are based on organizations outside health care. Many were developed to measure the quality of nursing care and are not appropriate for midwifery. There are, however, few models designed specifically for measuring midwifery care. Three methods for implementing quality in midwifery, are the *Monitor*, *Dynamic Standard Setting System* (DySSSy) and *Total Quality Management* (TQM).

Monitor

This method was developed from the Rush Medicus instrument, which originated in Chicago in the 1970s. It was adapted in the UK by Goldstone and Ball (Goldstone *et al.*, 1983) and uses external trained observers to monitor the quality of care as well as the quality of the environment. This is carried out by interviewing patients, and staff, by looking at records and by observing interactions between patients and nurses. *Midwifery Monitor* was developed from the original *Monitor* and incorporates a master checklist of quality-related criteria based on the results of consultation with midwives and studies concerned with assessing the quality of midwifery care. It is published in three volumes: *Pregnancy Care; Labour Care;* and *Post Natal Care* (Hughes and Goldstone, 1989). Standardized information is obtained about patient care and the environment and can be used for comparison purposes. However, implementing *Monitor* has cost implications, staff have no input into what is audited and the tool will not be sensitive to local variations in the service.

Royal College of Nursing Dynamic Standard Setting System

The Royal College of Nursing DySSSy was developed in the 1980s by Jane Clark and Helen Kendall and further developed by Professor Alison Kitson (Royal College of Nursing, 1990). It has its in roots in the *Standards of Care Project* (McFarlane, 1970) in the late 1960s, and has a 'bottom-up' approach. The system is characterized by small groups of nurses and midwives working together with a facilitator to set standards for their sphere of practice. The groups can be interprofessional. It is patient or client focused and a standardized format is used for writing standards based on Donabedian's (1966) structure, process and outcome. The standards are indexed so that standards in one area can be compared with those in another. It is important that this process is supported by managers at the top of the organization. The standards are ratified by the manager and are used to improve practice. They are audited regularly, preferably by those involved in setting the standards.

Health care settings that have successfully implemented DySSSy have been a good preparation for introducing TQM (Marr and Giebing, 1994).

Total Quality Management

Total Quality Management (TQM) is a philosophy that involves everyone in the organization in the quest for quality. It is based on the ideas of Deming and Juran in the 1950s and 1960s, and is a 'top-down' management-led approach. TQM has been defined as the system by which quality at each interface is assured. It is an approach to improving the effectiveness and flexibility of the service as a whole—a way of organising and involving the whole service, every authority, unit department, activity, every single person at every level to ensure that organised activities happen the way they are planned and seeking continuous improvement in performance' (Morris, 1989).

The idea behind TQM is that quality is 'managed' and not retrospectively corrected. The system is looked at as a whole, but each department is charged with looking at its service to make it more efficient and effective. This is achieved by staff commitment, management planning, empowering staff, appointing facilitators to go between management and staff groups, training, reducing variability and monitoring. The term total quality management is synonymous with *Continuous Quality Improvement* (CQI).

TQM is in its infancy in National Health Service hospitals in the UK. It remains to be seen whether it is a successful way of improving care in the maternity services or whether the way forward is through locally organized 'bottom-up' methods such as DySSSy or the similar approach described in this book.

Key points

- Quality is not a new idea.

- Evaluating the quality of health care, including midwifery care, is a relatively recent development.

- Florence Nightingale is acknowledged as the first person to systematically observe and evaluate outcomes of care and to implement change as a result.

- There are several approaches to implementing quality.

- The most widely used approach to quality health care is Donabedian's 'structure process outcome' (1966).

- Quality and audit issues are central to good midwifery practice.

References

Auld M. (1980) Midwifery standards. *Midwives Chronicle and Nursing Notes* January 1980: 5–11.

Bark P, Vincent C, Jones A, Savory J (1994) Clinical complaints: a means of improving quality of care. *Quality in Health Care* 3: 123–132.

Carter GB and Balme H (1936) Importance of evaluating care. In: Sale, D (1991) *Quality Assurance*. Macmillan: London.

Codman E (1914) The product of a hospital. *Surgery, Gynaecology and Obstetrics* 10: 491–494.

Cowell B and Wainwright D (1981) *Behind the Blue Door*. Baillière Tindall: London. p. 99.

Crombie I, Davies H, Abraham S and Florey C (1993) *The Audit Handbook Improving Health Care Through Clinical Audit*. John Wiley & Sons: Chichester.

Crosby P (1979) *Quality is Free: The Art of Making Quality Certain.* McGraw-Hill Book Co: New York. p. 17.

Dawson J (1993) The role of quality assurance in future midwifery practice. *Journal of Advanced Nursing* **18**: 1251–1258.

Department of Health (1989) *Working for Patients.* HMSO: London.

Department of Health (1991a) *Report of Confidential Enquiries into Maternal Deaths in the U.K. 1985–1987.* HMSO: London.

Department of Health (1991b) *Framework of Audit for Nursing Services.* HMSO: London. p.1.

Department of Health (1991c) *The Patient's Charter.* HMSO: London.

Department of Health (1993) *Changing Childbirth. Report of the Expert Maternity Group Part 1.* HMSO: London. p.64.

Department of Health (1996) *Complaints: Listening...Acting...Improving.* HMSO: London.

Donabedian A (1966) Evaluating the quality of medical care. *Millbank Memorial Fund Quarterly* **44**: 166–203.

Donabedian A (1970) Patient care evaluation. *Hospitals* April:131–136.

Donabedian A (1980) *Explorations in Quality Assessment and Monitoring Volume 1. The Definition of Quality and Approaches to its Assessment and Monitoring.* Health Administration Press: Michigan. p. 50.

Ellis R and Whittington D (1993) *Quality Assurance in Health Care, A Handbook.* Edward Arnold: London.

Firth-Cozens J (1996) Looking at effectiveness: ideas from the couch. *Quality in Health Care* **5**:55–59.

Frostick S, Radford P and Wallace W (1993) *Medical Audit Rationale and Practicalities.* University Press: Cambridge.

Goldstone LA, Ball JA and Collier M (1983) *Monitor. An index of the Quality of Nursing care for Acute Medical and Surgical Wards.* (Northern Staffing Levels Project) Newcastle upon Tyne Polytechnic Projects: Newcastle upon Tyne.

Groves EW (1908) A plea for uniform registration of operation results. *British Medical Journal* **ii**: 1008–1009.

Holy Bible (New International Version) Genesis i, 31. Hodder and Stoughton: London.

Hughes D and Goldstone L (1989) *Midwifery Monitor. Vol. I Pregnancy Care; Vol.II, Labour Care; Vol. III, Post Natal Care.* Poly Enterprises (Leeds) Ltd: Leeds.

Irvine D and Irvine S (1991) *Making Sense of Audit.* Radford Medical Press: Oxford. p.2.

King's Fund (1986) *Pursuing Quality. Independent Council for People with Mental Handicaps.* King's Fund: London.

Kitson A (1989) *Standards of Care: A Framework for Quality.* Royal College of Nursing: London.

Lee R and Jones L (1933) *The Fundamentals of Good Medical Care.* University of Chicago Press: Chicago.

The Little Oxford Dictionary (1980). Oxford University Press: Oxford.

Maresh M (1994) *Audit in Obstetrics and Gynaecology.* Blackwell Scientific Publications: Oxford. p. 4.

Marr H and Giebing H (1994) *Quality in Nursing.* Campion Press: Edinburgh. p. 14.

Maxwell RJ (1984) Quality assessment in health. *British Medical Journal* **288**: 1470–1472.

McFarlane J (1970) *The Proper Study of the Nurse: RCN Standards of Nursing Care.* Royal College of Nursing: London.

Morris B (1989) Total quality management. *International Journal of Health Care Quality Assurance* **2**(3): 4–6.

Nightingale F (1863) Notes on hospitals. In: Rosenbury (ed.) (1989) *Florence Nightingale on Hospital Reform.* Garland Publishing: New York. p. 45.

Ovretveit J (1992) *Health Service Quality. An Introduction to Quality Methods for Health Services.* Blackwell Scientific Publications: Oxford. p. 1.

Pirsig R (1974) *Zen and the Art of Motor Cycle Maintenance.* Corgi: London.

Royal College of Obstetricians and Gynaecologists (1995) *Report of the Audit Committee's Group on Communication Standards in Obstetrics.* RCOG: London. p. 4.

Royal College of Nursing (1990) *Quality Patient Care: An Introduction to the RCN Dynamic Standard Setting System (DySSSy).* Scutari Press: London.

Royal College of Nursing (1991) *Standards of Care: Midwifery.* Royal College of Nursing: London.

Sale D (1991) *Quality Assurance.* Macmillan: London. p. 1.

Stewart I (1919) Possibilities of standardization of nursing techniques. *Modern Hospital* **12**(6): 451–454. In: Sale D (1991) *Quality Assurance.* Macmillan: London.

Shaw C (1987) *Introducing Quality Assurance.* Kings Fund: London. p. 11.

Shaw C (1992) The background. In: Smith R (ed.) *Audit in Action.* British Medical Journal: London. p.4.

Smith R (1992) Audit and research. *British Medical Journal* **305**: 905–906.

United Kingdom Central Council for Nursing, Midwifery and Health Visiting (1994) *The Midwife's Code of Practice.* UKCC: London. p.3.

Walshe K, Coles J (1993) *Evaluating Audit. Developing a Framework.* CASPE Research: London. p. 22.

Williamson JW (1978) Formulating priorities for quality assurance activity: description of a method and its application. *Journal of the American Medical Association* **239**: 631–637.

Wilson CRM (1987) *Hospital-Wide Quality Assurance.* WB Saunders Co., Canada Ltd: Toronto. p. 8.

World Health Organization (1985) *Targets of Health for All.* World Health Organization Regional Office for Europe: Copenhagen.

2 Standards, Audits and Quality Cycles

Quality cycles

Implementing quality is a never-ending process of evaluation, action and re-evaluation. It is a process, not an event. The process has been described as a 'quality cycle' by Lang (1976), emphasizing the continual process of setting standards, auditing and implementing change. The term 'spiral' (Bucknall *et al.*, 1992) has been used more recently, indicating the 'progress' as well as the 'process' of change. There are many types and variations of quality cycles, some are complex. However, the principles of implementing quality are simple and are summarized in *Figure 2.1*.

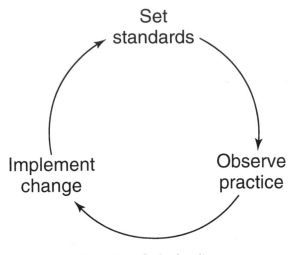

Figure 2.1   *Cycle of quality*

Setting standards

Setting standards, as discussed in Chapter 1, is not a new idea. Every day, we measure events against standards we have already set for ourselves. We do it without thinking. Where we shop is usually decided by our standards and our previous experience measured against those standards. When we enter a store for the first time, we make judgements about the atmosphere, cleanliness, service and the goods on offer. And we continue to measure our experience against what we have come to expect. Where we eat out usually depends on our previous experience or the recommendation of others, whose judgements we subject to our own tests—do they like the same food? do they demand the same standards of service? do they spend roughly the same amount of money as we do?

The standards of service we expect often vary according to where we are, who we are with and how great our need is. When travelling in a remote region of the world we may lower our standards, depending on how desperate we are for the service! Standards are not 'written in stone' and we may suspend our usual standards in unusual or urgent situations and adopt them again later when the crisis has passed.

This 'standard setting' is, of course, carried out largely subconsciously and starts at an early age as our personalities develop and we start to evolve our own likes and dislikes.

Our lives, then, are governed by a set of dynamic standards, which evolve with different situations and changing tastes, and are an everyday part of life for everybody. Setting professional standards is similar.

When setting professional standards, the question needs to be asked 'Where do we want to be?' There does not necessarily need to be an identified 'problem' (though this is often the case) to set standards. There may simply be a need to improve a good service or to put such a service on a more organized or formal footing in order to be able to audit it and make improvements when appropriate. Standard statements have been defined as 'professionally agreed levels of performance appropriate to the population addressed which reflect what is acceptable, achievable, observable and measurable' (Sale, 1991). Setting standards is the subject of Chapter 4.

Observing practice

'Observing practice' simply refers to the audit process of comparing practice against the standard. It asks the question 'Where are we now?' In everyday terms it is illustrated by going into a shop and measuring the service against our expectations. How we actually measure the service will vary. One way would be to measure the time we wait to be served. Another way would be the subjective impression we form as we see queues of people waiting to be served. Yet another way may be by how others judge the service: hearing complaints from other customers may influence our views. We use these sorts of methods all the time to 'audit' the services we receive everyday. They do not differ much from those used to carry out a clinical audit.

An clinical example might be the waiting times in an antenatal clinic. Mothers may have to wait a long time before being seen. This could be concluded from a formal audit based on a standard that has already been set (in this case *The Patient's Charter* standard (Department of Health (1991)) and measuring the periods of time spent waiting. Alternatively it may be concluded anecdotally, i.e. seeing crowds of mothers waiting in clinics and concluding that there is a problem with long waiting times. Finally, the problem may emerge because a mother makes a official complaint about being kept waiting too long. Carrying out audits and making sense of audit results are addressed in Chapters 4 and 6.

Implementing change

In terms of the quality cycle, implementing change is about asking the question 'what do we need to do in order to get where we want to be?' There is little point in setting standards and auditing them if appropriate changes are not then made. Chapter 7 considers how to implement change in response to audit results.

Auditing care

Avedis Donabedian first articulated the idea that medical care could be evaluated by auditing structure, process and outcome in his famous 1966 paper. He suggested that process and outcome in particular were key indicators of a service. The foundations of high quality care, he maintained, are standards of good clinical practice.

Standards were defined by Donabedian as 'the extent of agreement concerning facts and values within the profession...' and that they ' ...are set by standard textbooks or publications, panels of physicians, highly qualified practitioners...' (Donabedian, 1966). A 'standard' has been further defined as the 'optimum level of care against which performance is compared' (Gallant and McLane, 1979) and an 'agreed upon level of excellence' (Lang, 1976).

Ideally standards are dynamic, not static. They exist as benchmarks of the service, but may be improved and refined with time.

The concept of setting standards by the 'structure, process, outcome' model was developed on the basis of Donabedian's work and the ideas expanded in this book are based on this model.

Structure

Structure refers to the resources needed to attain the standard. These may consist of buildings, rooms, services, personnel (adequate staffing levels may be alluded to here), existing policies and procedures, professional guidelines and Unit policies. Other resources may include literature, leaflets and videos.

Process

Process refers to what is to be done, by whom, when and how, with the resources to achieve the standard. It may include techniques or interventions. It is not, however, a detailed description of procedures.

Outcome

Outcome refers to what 'comes out' of the combination

of structure and process, the 'end result of care' (Ellis and Whittingon, 1993). It is the desired result. For example 'mothers are sutured within one hour of normal delivery,' 'all babies are given vitamin K with the verbal consent of the mother or father.' Outcomes need to be specific, measurable and attainable, and should relate closely to the standard statement.

Monitoring Tools

Monitoring tools are used to monitor or audit the standard. Donabedian (1966) suggested that care could be evaluated in several ways: examining clinical records, direct observation and eliciting others' (fellow clinicians' or consumers') views. These methods are all used as audit methods today, although the latter is probably used most commonly.

Questionnaires. These consist of written questions, which are given to people in a particular sample for completion. Their success depends on the people in the sample being literate and highly motivated to complete them, the questions being unambiguous and there being a pen to hand! They are relatively cheap and quick to administer, anonymous and are easy to analyse if closed questions are used. However, response rates may be low and those not returning questionnaires may not be representative of those who do. Some questions may be misunderstood or not completed.

Interview schedules. These are used when people are interviewed and asked for their opinions. Responses are written down by the interviewer. The response rate tends to be higher than with questionnaires, but it is of limited value for people whose first language is not English unless a translator is available. Interviewing is a skill that needs to be understood by the interviewer.

Respondents may feel pressured to give a 'right' answer and may be influenced by the interviewer. It may also be expensive on time and manpower.

Examining clinical records. The review of clinical records whether handwritten or computerized can be an effective audit tool. It may be used to monitor certain recorded data or the completeness or comprehensiveness of the documentation itself. Accessing records, however, may be difficult or time-consuming.

Direct observation. This can be used as a method to actually 'see' what is happening. It is, however, expensive in terms of time and resources, the observer may need training and people who are being observed may alter their behaviour, the so-called Hawthorne effect.

In Practice Some Standards are Easier to Measure than Others

Measuring waiting times is relatively easy, but measuring attitudes (e.g. satisfaction) in a way that is valid and replicable is harder. And how can we measure the information given to a mother? Do we ask the midwife what information she gave, opening up the possibility of bias? Or do we ask the mother whether she was given the information, knowing she may have forgotten a perfectly adequate explanation given some time ago? Or do we audit both, and then which result will be the most valid? As discussed above, all audit tools have their limitations. The practicalities of how to use the resources, personnel and time available are important factors, and the appropriate monitoring tool will usually be a trade-off between what is ideal and what is possible within existing resources.

The practicalities of setting standards and developing monitoring tools are expanded in Chapter 4.

Key points

- Everybody subconsciously sets standards all the time and monitors (or audits) their experience against their expectations.

- The 'quality cycle' contains three main principles: setting standards, comparing practice with expectation (audit) and implementing change.

- Donabedian first suggested evaluating the quality of clinical care by breaking down the components of care into structure, process and outcome. His ideas have been developed and this method of evaluating care is widely used.

References

Bucknall C, Robertson C, Moran F and Stevenson R (1992) Improving management of asthma: closing the loop or progressing along the audit spiral? *Health Care* 1:15.

Department of Health (1991) *The Patient's Charter.* HMSO: London.

Donabedian A (1996) Evaluating the quality of medical care. *Millbank Memorial Fund Quarterly* 44:166.

Ellis R and Whittington D (1993) *Quality Assurance in Health Care. A Handbook.* Edward Arnold: London. p. 21.

Gallant B and McLane A (1979) Outcome criteria – a process for validation at unit level. *Journal of Nursing and Administration* 9:14.

Lang N (1976) *Issues in Quality Assurance in Nursing.* ANA Issues in Evaluative Research. American Nursing Association.

Sale D (1991) *Quality Assurance.* Macmillan Education Ltd: London. p. 54.

Section 2 Implementing Quality

3 Setting the Scene

Having the desire to implement quality initiatives in a maternity service is admirable. The desire alone is not enough to ensure success, but certain 'key principles', however, will ensure the success of a quality improvement programme.

Quality strategy

For the concept of quality improvement to succeed, it needs to be built into the 'fabric' of the organization, be it the hospital, community unit or maternity unit. One way of doing this is to produce a mission statement or philosophy of care in which quality assurance is implicit. Many hospitals and units have included some sort of quality strategy into their mission statements or philosophies of care. Professional bodies have also produced similar statements, which can be used as a focus to implement quality improvements. The Royal College of Midwives issued the following philosophy of care in 1992:

'The aim of the midwifery profession is to provide a service which facilitates the safe and satisfying transition of women to motherhood. This is achieved principally by the processes of supporting, caring, guiding, monitoring and educating. The unique and personal needs of women in their childbearing years are central to this service.'

The philosophy of midwifery care may be stated as a set of aims as shown by the following example from the Nottingham City Hospital Maternity Unit:

'To improve continuity of care, to identify individual needs and give a more personalized service, to increase the mother's satisfaction with her care, to enable midwives to retain and develop their midwifery skills, to enable midwives to fulfil their complete role and thus improve job satisfaction and to develop staff for a more efficient and effectively run service.'

Mission statements are often used to encapsulate a unit's aims and objectives as shown by this example from Derby City General Hospital (1993), which states that their midwifery service is about:

'Entering into partnership with the mother, providing education and guidance, supporting informed decisions throughout pregnancy, childbirth and parenthood.'

Other elements of their mission statement refer to:

'providing a holistic approach to care, using resources effectively, continuity of care, cooperating with other health professionals, being honest about the quality of care provided and reducing morbidity and mortality rates.'

Mission statements and philosophies of care, if properly used, have the advantage of focusing minds and thus, hopefully, care by providing aims that everybody in the organization aspires to. This is the ideal. Unfortunately, the existence of a mission statement does not guarantee high quality of care. It is only a starting point, an 'umbrella' under which all quality issues should be related and focused.

It has been suggested by Sale (1991) that producing a philosophy of care should be the first task of a quality or standard setting group. However, to avoid reinventing the wheel, it should be ascertained whether a philosophy of care already exists in the organization or whether the one produced by the Royal College of Midwives, for example, can be accepted or adapted for use in the particular unit. It is time consuming to produce mission statements and philosophies of care and it is probably better for quality groups to concentrate on setting clinical standards of care.

The midwifery manager

It has already been said that, although a quality strategy is important, it is not a guarantee of a quality service. What matters more is that the manager of a unit positively and enthusiastically supports the concept of quality improvement and is willing to make the manpower and resources available so that the system can be set up and maintained. 'Nodding agreement' is not enough. Without immediate and continuing management support and interest, enthusiasm will wane and the impetus will be lost. Lack of support has been found to be a major reason for the failure of standard setting groups (Moss, 1995). Management support and encouragement are two of the most important ingredients of a successful quality implementation programme.

The other important responsibilities of the manager are to feed down changes in unit policy that involve quality issues, to contribute ideas and feedback to the groups, and to ratify by signature the standards produced by the standard setting groups. This makes the standards part of the unit policy.

Another valuable part of the manager's role is to inform other senior colleagues in the organization of the work carried out by the quality groups, so encouraging awareness of quality issues and dissemination of ideas in other units.

The quality coordinator

The quality coordinator is another important key player in the success of a quality improvement programme. Though clinical standards of care are produced by the standard setting groups, these groups cannot run themselves. Staff who are involved in standard setting groups as well as giving care to mothers and babies cannot be expected to be able to coordinate groups, organize meetings, liaise with other health professionals and organize audits. This is the job of the coordinator.

A senior midwife should be given the job of setting up and coordinating quality groups and implementing quality improvements in the unit. This can be either on a part-time or full-time basis. The coordinator should be a clinically experienced midwife who has an interest in quality issues and is able to network and negotiate confidently with other disciplines and departments, i.e. medical staff, neonatal unit staff, medical physics, medical records staff, laboratory staff and estates departments. She or he should have the interpersonal skills that enable the organization and facilitation of groups. The ability to enable group members to participate freely, not allowing hierarchies in the group and not allowing strong personalities to dominate is very important. The coordinator will also need to have the skills and maturity to guide discussion to prevent 'red herrings' taking over discussions and to be able to go along with majority decisions.

Some knowledge of quality issues is of course essential and many hospitals and units run courses on standard setting. In addition, the quality coordinator should preferably have some training in audit or research methods and to be able to analyse and present data in a methodical way. It is vital to argue a case from facts, not feelings, and present a strong case that gains the respect of other colleagues and disciplines.

Many hospitals and units run courses on audit and a variety of other courses, which include learning about and developing the skill of facilitating groups. The English National Board (ENB) course 870 on research is a useful course for the quality coordinator.

The main duties of the quality coordinator are shown in *Box 3.1*. Perhaps most importantly, the quality coordinator needs to have a commitment and enthusiasm for quality improvement, a desire to see the service to mothers and babies improved, and a willingness and ability to persuade colleagues to work together to achieve this aim.

Group members

Which staff should be involved in standard setting in midwifery? Should there be just midwives, or should there be representatives from all disciplines who are likely to be involved in setting maternity standards? A case can be made for both uni- and multidisciplinary groups. There are advantages and disadvantages for both.

Undisciplinary groups (i.e. midwives only) are able to see midwifery issues clearly, but may be too narrowly focused and run the danger of lack of cooperation from other disciplines. An example of this would be a group looking at standardizing the interpretation

Box 3.1   Duties of the quality coordinator

- Setting up quality groups

- Organizing staff training

- Organizing meetings

- Organizing the typing of minutes, drafts of standards, audit reports

- Liaising with other health professionals and departments

- Getting feedback from colleagues

- Organizing audits

- Communicating with staff about the purposes of the audits and providing information and resources

- Collating and analysing data

- Presenting audit findings formally in reports

- Presenting audit findings verbally on an informal basis to staff (e.g. in meetings, presentations)

of cardiotocographs (CTGs). Clearly, in this case obstetricians need to be involved.

Groups that are too broadly focused, however, though they involve other disciplines, run the danger of waning interest if standards are discussed and set that do not involve a particular discipline. An example of this would be involving obstetricians on a standard for breastfeeding on maternity wards.

In practice few standards are purely 'midwifery' orientated. Most encroach onto other areas of practice. One solution is to have a 'core' group of midwives, maybe based in a particular area of practice, e.g. antenatal clinic or postnatal ward, and possibly an auxiliary and a receptionist and invite others to attend meetings on an ad hoc basis when the particular standard under discussion demands their expertise. An example of this would be a standard on giving information about vitamin K to mothers. A paediatrician could be invited to contribute to the discussion about what needs to be communicated verbally and what needs to go into written information. This fosters positive links with other disciplines and departments, enables a broader view to be taken into account, and is vital in communicating the same standard information to mothers. When drafting a standard on waiting times in antenatal clinic it makes sense to involve a member of medical records staff because any discussion of waiting times is bound to cover the subject of spacing of appointment times. A standard involving ethnic issues should involve an interpreter if there is one who can contribute his or her perspective on communicating to ethnic minorities.

Other groups may be set up around a particular standard, rather than an area of practice, e.g. interpreting CTGs. Once the standard has been set and implemented, the group may be disbanded and other groups set up to look at other subjects.

All midwifery staff need to be given the opportunity to be involved in standard setting. Many midwives will have a particular area or subject of interest and this should be respected where possible when the groups are formed. Ideally there should be a mixture of senior and junior staff in each group so that the group benefits from both experience and newer ideas.

Receptionists and auxiliaries work closely with mothers

and babies and are an important part of the workforce with a unique view and role. They should also be given the opportunity to be involved in standard setting.

Doctors also have an interest in standards in maternity care and should be offered the opportunity of participating in groups. Senior house officers tend to be appointed for only short periods of time. However, registrars and consultants, and in health centres, general practitioners, may well be interested in joining a group that looks at a subject requiring their expertise as well as that of midwives (e.g. cardiotocograph interpretation, postnatal haemoglobins, obstetric emergencies).

It is helpful to have lay members in standard setting groups where this is appropriate. Mothers who have been consumers of the service also have a unique view and can contribute valuable insights about how it feels to be on the other end of the service. Appropriate topics for consumer input may be privacy and dignity, support with breast feeding, and information provision. One way of involving lay members may be to ask members of the local National Childbirth Trust group whether any members would be interested in joining.

Training

Training needs to be given to staff. The principles of standard setting are simple, but it is useful for staff to attend a teaching session to 'try out' setting a standard themselves and to see how standards work in practice by hearing about successful examples. Training days may be run by hospital quality departments, midwifery education departments or the quality coordinator.

Autonomy

It is important that the groups have autonomy. They should not simply be the mouthpiece of the manager, otherwise they will lose credibility. Group members need to have the freedom to choose a topic or standard that they feel is most relevant. Their ideas and suggestions will no doubt be modified by feedback from others (including the manager), but the group must be allowed to run its own affairs whilst remaining accountable to the Midwifery Manager.

'Time out'

Time out should be given for group members to be able to meet together. This is vital if quality initiatives are to take root and also demonstrates the commitment of the organization and the manager to quality. This need only be about one hour every 3–4 weeks. The overlap between shifts is often a good time to meet and is an effective use of time.

Perhaps most importantly each group member should have a commitment to the group, to attend meetings and to provide feedback from their ward or department areas to the group. Members need to be told at the beginning that this is the basis of the group and asked to agree to it.

Quality circles should not be seen either as secret societies or elitist groups. The members should view themselves as representatives of other midwives in their ward or team, and keep their particular ward, department or team informed about what is going on.

All maternity staff

All staff involved in the care of mothers and babies need to be able to have the opportunity to feed back and comment on proposed standards and to have access to audit results. Feedback can be given through group members or by being able to write comments on draft standards.

Audit results should be made available to staff by written reports, information posters put up on notice boards in coffee rooms, staff rooms and offices, and by verbal presentations from the quality coordinator.

It is only fair that feedback is given to those who have contributed to the production of standards and audits. Demonstrated improvements in the service are the result of many people's efforts and this needs to be acknowledged.

Key points

- It is important, though not essential, that the unit has a mission statement or agreed philosophy of care to act as a focus for quality improvement initiatives.

- It is essential that the midwifery manager demonstrates a commitment to and takes a positive and continued interest in quality improvement and commits resources and time to allow standard setting groups to be set up.

- A quality coordinator should be appointed, part or full-time, who is a senior clinician, with research or audit training and the ability to coordinate and facilitate groups.

- All maternity unit staff should be given the opportunity to be involved in standard setting groups and should be able to give feedback and have access to audit results.

- It is important to train interested staff in the principles of standard setting.

- Group autonomy and 'time out' are vital for a group's success.

References

Derby City General Hospital (1993). *Maternity Standards.*

Moss E (1995). *An Evolution of Standard Setting in an Acute Provider Unit.* Unpublished dissertation for M.Sc. in Quality in Health and Social Care, University of Leeds.

Sale D (1991) *Quality Assurance.* Macmillan Education Ltd: London. p. 4.

4 Setting up Quality Groups

The scene is set. The midwifery manager is enthusiastic about delivering quality to mothers and babies, has a positive commitment to implementing quality and has appointed a quality coordinator to facilitate change. She or he is willing to commit resources for staff training, and time out for group members to meet in autonomous groups. There may or may not be a mission statement or philosophy of care, but there will be a commitment to change and implementing quality in the organization.

Staff may be recruited in different ways, depending on the size of the unit or team. Approaches may be made individually if the team is small. In larger units, a letter could be sent to all staff, either from the midwifery manager or the quality coordinator. Posters are also a good way of recruiting people. Some training in quality issues should be organized for recruits. It is important that prospective group members are told that the commitment to groups is important (i.e. attendance at meetings where possible and getting feedback from colleagues). It is also important that group members should be volunteers. There is no place for people who have been 'volunteered' or who are reluctant members, for whatever reason.

The groups may be set up in several ways depending on the number of people interested, the size of the unit, and the time available to the quality coordinator. Obviously, a full-time quality coordinator will be able to take on more groups than one who is part time.

One option is to start with one group and to set standards on subjects related to midwifery care. If a lot of people are interested, several groups can be set up simultaneously, each representing a different ward or area in care. Groups can be made up of representatives from different wards or 'teams' and set up around various areas in the maternity unit (e.g. labour suite, antenatal clinic and wards). A further differentiation can be made for the wards between care of mothers and care of babies. Standards can then be set relating to these areas. This has been found to be a very successful approach.

To avoid fragmentation between areas, a broader approach is more appropriate for some unit-wide issues (e.g. security, stillbirth, ethnic issues and interpretation of cardiotocographs).

Small groups generally work well if they are made up of 6–12 people. If the group is too small, ideas and 'cross-fertilization' of ideas may not be produced in the same way as in larger groups. If the group is too big it becomes impersonal and some members may feel inhibited. Having said this, it is rare to have a full complement of group members for a variety of reasons such as clinical duties, and shift changes. It is therefore wise to aim where possible for two representatives from teams so that there is continuity.

All groups need a leader. This can be either the quality coordinator or an appointed leader. A leader may 'emerge' after time as someone who has leadership qualities and is respected by the group. She or he is responsible for facilitating discussion, making sure that each group member has their say, keeping the discussion focused, and making sure the meetings are minuted.

Meetings should take place in a room where members are unlikely to be disturbed, away from telephones and clinical demands. Offering coffee or tea or making the meeting a working lunch may encourage group attendance. Providing cake or biscuits on occasion can do wonders for group 'ambience'!

The first meeting

The first meeting should consist of introductions where necessary and a short general introduction by the quality coordinator about quality and what it is hoped will be achieved. If training has not already been provided, it should be made clear that it will. The basis of the group should be reiterated (i.e. everyone has something to offer and therefore a part to play). Hierarchies are not encouraged, but an open atmosphere that encourages discussion and an exchange of ideas is. Differences of opinion are inevitable, but standards which will improve patient care are the aim, and this will be achieved by discussion, an exploration of issues, and consensus. Commitment to the group is important. Members should attend meetings if possible, and send apologies if not. Getting feedback from colleagues is also an important role of group members. Members should be informed that meetings will normally last for one hour, so that they know they will not be trapped in meetings that go on too long.

Minutes of meetings should be taken by one member of the group, preferably not the leader. This is the formal record of the meeting. Minute taking can be rotated around the group unless one person wants to take on the job.

A discussion should then be held about what is thought to be a suitable topic around which to set the first standard. If the group is based around a particular clinical area (e.g. postnatal care) then the topics should centre on this. Although standards do not have to be set around a particular 'problem', in practice they often are. Ideas for topics for standards may be taken from The Patient's Charter (Department of Health, 1991), comments from mothers, suggestions from staff, or recommendations made by professional bodies such as the United Kingdom Central Council for Nursing, Midwifery and Health Visiting or the Royal College of Midwives, or outside bodies such as the Audit Commission, the Community Health Council or the King's Fund. Suggested ideas for standards are listed in *Box 4.1*.

Box 4.1   *Ideas for standards*

Patients' Charter standards

- Privacy and dignity

- Ethnic issues

- Clinic waiting times

- Named midwife

Midwifery practice

- Improving breastfeeding rates

- Care of mothers who have a fetal loss or stillbirth

- Interpreting cardiotocographs

(continued overleaf)

Box 4.1   Ideas for standards (continued)

Information to mothers

- Blood tests in pregnancy

- Screening tests in pregnancy

- Smoking in pregnancy

- Amniocentesis

- Vitamin K

- Tube feeding babies

- Reducing the risk of cot death

- Guthrie test

- Jaundice

- Security

- Postnatal exercises

- Bottle feed preparation

- Orientation to the ward

One way of generating ideas for standards is by brainstorming. This is a method that encourages a free flow of ideas by each member who contributes ideas about what she or he thinks are areas to address (*Box 4.2*).

After everyone has had a chance to contribute, ideas should be grouped into categories. A consensus will usually emerge about what is a suitable topic to concentrate on.

Box 4.2 Brainstorming

- One idea at a time

- Allow all ideas

- No criticisms or ridicule

- Write all ideas on flip chart or white board

- Allow silences for people to think

- Encourage everyone to contribute

Only one standard should be worked on at a time. It is better to start small than to be too ambitious. Taking on a standard such as interpreting cardiotocographs, for example, is a large project. A small easily contained standard that is confined to a particular area such as information to mothers about vitamin K or blood tests in pregnancy is an appropriate starter.

The meeting should end at the agreed time, even if no particular decisions have been made, and the business deferred until the next meeting. Meetings should normally be held every 3–4 weeks. The dates of the next two meetings should be fixed so that off-duty requests can be made well in advance.

Subsequent meetings

Producing Standards

At subsequent meetings discussion will continue on the

chosen topic and a standard statement, structure, process, outcome and monitoring tool will be decided. This can be a lengthy process and can take several meetings over several months. An example of a standard illustrating the different components is given in *Box 4.3*.

The Standard Statement

A standard statement should be relevant, understandable, measurable, behavioural and achievable, i.e. RUMBA (Wilson 1987). It should also be professionally agreed, unambiguous and be one sentence containing one main idea.

Structure

As discussed in Chapter 2, the structure consists of the resources needed to fulfil the standard. This will usually include personnel, policies and procedures already in existence. It may also include the areas or rooms needed to attain a standard. Where further resources are needed innovative ways of using wasted resources can sometimes be found. Setting standards does not always have to cost money. In fact, unnecessary routines can sometimes be eliminated or adapted to accommodate the resources needed.

Some standards will require extra resources. For a standard on privacy and dignity, it may be decided for example that curtains or 'Do Not Enter' signs are needed. Having professionally agreed that a standard needs to be met, there is a strong case for the manager to provide the resources to meet the standard.

Many standards involve information giving to supplement verbal explanations. If satisfactory leaflets are already in existence, they should be used. Designing leaflets is time consuming and has resource implications.

Many excellent leaflets are produced (sometimes free) by bodies such as the Health Education Authority or specialist organizations such as The Toxoplasmosis Trust, the National Asthma Campaign and local groups involved in giving information to people with thalassaemia or sickle cell disease. There is no point in reinventing the wheel. However, appropriate leaflets may not be available or information may be needed to reflect a particular unit's policy on a subject (e.g. security or ward information). It is then necessary to design 'in house' leaflets. These are relatively easy to produce if access to a computer is available with the appropriate software. The group discusses what needs to go into the leaflet and a group member may offer to put the ideas together. If the quality coordinator has the skills and access to appropriate equipment, he or she can then make a copy of the leaflet (or persuade somebody else to!) for comments and feedback.

Leaflets should look attractive, and be printed or well reproduced (no photocopies of photocopies!) and their supply should be well organized. An original may be given to the receptionist to photocopy when supplies run low. If the leaflet is a ward information leaflet, laminated copies may be considered to go by every bedside so that they can be used by successive mothers during their hospital stay.

Teaching sessions may be needed to achieve some standards. Who is going to provide them? Will they need financing? Often specialist staff can be persuaded to give talks or training sessions on subjects such as cot death, haemorrhagic disease, perineal suturing, and siting of intravenous cannulae within the unit. Details like this need to be thought through carefully when the standard is being drafted.

Process

Who is going to do what and when? The details need to

be thought through carefully. The standard will stand or fall on how effectively the 'people' element works. The process needs to work in the real world. For example, in a standard involving giving leaflets to mothers, who will keep the leaflet stocks topped up? Who will give a particular leaflet to the mother? The doctor, midwife or auxiliary? Does it matter? What may be more important in some situations is that the mother gets the information, rather than who hands it to her. In other cases it may be seen as an important part of the midwife's role that the midwife gives out a particular leaflet as an adjunct to verbal information. These issues need careful thought, discussion and agreement from all those involved in implementing the standard.

Outcome

The outcome should be a reflection of the standard statement. For example, 'mothers are seen within 30 minutes of their appointment times'. However, it may not always be possible to measure direct outcomes. What may need to be measured is an aspect of the process. For example, for a standard on giving mothers information on how to reduce the risk of cot death, an outcome measure could be that all mothers are given the Department of Health leaflet. Another outcome measure could be that mothers know specifically what they can do to reduce the risk of cot death.

Monitoring tools

All standards need a monitoring tool, and all outcome criteria should be measured. The most common ways of auditing standards are asking questions, examining records, or direct observation.

Asking Questions

Simply making an outcome measure a question is often an effective and simple way of monitoring a standard. For example the standard statement 'Mothers will understand the reason for amniocentesis' (outcome measure) can be turned into 'Did you understand the reason for your amniocentesis?' (monitoring tool). Other information may also be asked for. For example, was the mother was given an information leaflet? Did she find it helpful? There is no reason why information that is not necessarily in the standard cannot be elicited (e.g. whether the mother is a multipara or primipara, which clinic she attended, which ward she was on and other comments that may be made by the mother). Analysing this sort of information may cast light on different practices and show up weak areas. Staff may also be asked questions.

Interview or questionnaire? It needs to be decided whether the questions should be put in an interview or questionnaire format. There are advantages and disadvantages to both methods as discussed in Chapter 2.

Questionnaires are useful audit tools in leaflets. The mother can then answer the questions and return the form. This is especially useful when leaflets are given to mothers to take home with them (e.g. amniocentesis information). Another situation is in clinic when waiting times need to be measured. The mother is given a form on arrival and asked to complete the appointment time, arrival time and 'time first seen.' The form is handed in on the way home.

Examining Records

It may be possible to monitor standards by auditing records: for example, monitoring delivery–suturing time intervals by accessing the maternity computer database. Simple calculations of how long mothers waited to be sutured can then be made either manually or by a computer program. Supplementary information can be obtained by building in a questionnaire to be displayed on screen at an appropriate place during data input into the computer asking for reasons for any delay and giving options with yes/no or free text answers.

Mothers' casenotes can be audited to see if records have been completed. Other records may also be examined such as delivery records, incident books, and diaries.

Waiting times in clinic have been monitored successfully by a 'bar coding' method. Staff at various stages in the clinic have a handheld bar code 'swiper,' which is used to swipe a card held by patients going through the various stages of clinics. The information is then held on a database for analysis.

Direct Observation

Standards can be monitored by direct observation. To audit a standard on welcoming mothers for example, a member of staff may be delegated to observe staff and mother interactions and note whether the mother was welcomed with a smile, how she was addressed, and whether direct eye contact took place. As mentioned in Chapter 2, this is a time-consuming audit method, staff need to be trained in observation techniques, and there may be a Hawthorne effect (when the behaviour of people being observed changes, as an effect of being observed).

Choice of monitoring tool

Each monitoring tool needs to be thought through individually, but often the easiest method is an interview schedule, particularly if there are several standards to audit. High response rates can be achieved and those who cannot read or write are not at a disadvantage.

Pre-Standard Audits

Sometimes it may be decided to carry out an audit before a standard is set, perhaps to find out whether there is a problem and what its extent is. The results are useful as comparisons can be made with this 'baseline data' when subsequent audits are carried out.

Timing

Timing of audits needs to be discussed. Asking a mother if she is satisfied with her care when she is attached to an intravenous infusion after a caesarian section is likely to produce a positive answer! On the other hand, asking the mother questions by interview or questionnaire when she has gone home may elicit more valid responses, but would be impractical and have huge resource and organizational implications. One compromise is to ask the mother questions at discharge. Mothers should always be told that the questionnaires or interviews are anonymous and given the option of declining to participate.

The group also needs to decide how often the standard needs to be monitored. Standards may be monitored more often at first (e.g. three- or six-monthly), particularly if there has been a problem, and then annually. When a few standards have been set, it may be more practical to monitor them together to avoid 'survey fatigue' among staff.

Sample Size and Characteristics

When carrying out audits it needs to be decided

whether every person in the particular population needs to be audited (a census) or just a sample. If, for example, the population to be sampled are mothers having an amniocentesis, then, as this is a relatively uncommon procedure, it may be decided to monitor every mother who has an amniocentesis over a period of time, say one year. However, if the sample population is hospital antenatal clinic attenders, then clearly it would not be feasible or desirable to audit all visits in one year. An acceptable sample of 400 patients per quarter when monitoring Patient's Charter standards for outpatients has been suggested (Department of Health, 1993).

How big should the sample be? This is a common question and here, as in many other areas, the answer is a trade-off between the ideal and the possible, given the limited time and resources. It is a common misconception that the bigger the sample size the more accurate the results. The size of sample does need to be big enough to give results that are valid, and there are problems with large samples. The larger the sample, the more mistakes occur due to 'survey fatigue' and the difficulties in handling a large amount of data. Large samples are also time consuming to analyse. However, there are problems, with small samples. Very small audits will not provide results that can be generalized to a larger population. As a rule of thumb, a sample of around 100 participants will give results that can reasonably be assumed to be valid. For a large annual audit 3–4 weeks' of data should be collected.

Another issue to be considered is whether the sample is representative, meaning two things: that the sample represents a cross-section of the relevant population and certain groups are not excluded; and that the sample is as complete as possible (i.e. as many mothers as possible in the chosen sample are represented).

There are many different methods of sampling, and explanations of these are outside the scope of this book. Recommended books on statistics that include information about sampling techniques are Clegg (1990), Kirk and Miller (1986) and Rowntree (1981). However, the characteristics of the sampling frame need to be clear (e.g. postnatal mothers at discharge, mothers who are sutured after normal delivery, mothers admitted for routine induction). If exclusions are to be made (e.g. mothers whose baby is on the neonatal unit or whose baby has died), these need to be made clear. 'Atypical' periods such as Christmas and bank holidays should be avoided when carrying out an audit, as workload may be unusually low (or high!) and this may bias the results.

When the audit is carried out, it is important that it is systematic and that the data sets are as complete as possible. The more missing data there are the less the results can be relied on to be accurate, and this can seriously bias the results. A 70% response rate is generally thought to be reasonably representative. If possible, where data are missing it is important that the reasons for non- or part-completion are taken into consideration (e.g. ethnicity, illiteracy, refusal). One reason why data may be missing is that questions are ambiguous. For this reason it is important to carry out a pilot study to test out the monitoring tool. In this way, ambiguous questions or methods can be modified.

For some audits, collecting a whole year's data will be no problem if the data are on a computer. One year of data on postnatal haemoglobin concentrations, for example, is easy to obtain if they are stored on a database and are accessible to clinicians. These data will give an accurate picture of how many are carried out and the levels, if the data sets are reasonably complete. However, as mentioned above, missing data may have particular characteristics; in this case those who went home early and did not therefore have a haemoglobin test probably had a normal haemoglobin concentration so the results could be biased and tend to represent more abnormal haemoglobin concentrations.

It may be claimed that audits are less rigorous than research. However, this does not mean that audit results are necessarily less valid or reliable (Kirk and Miller, 1986).

The draft standard

After the standard statement, resources, process, outcome and monitoring tool have been decided, they are typed up in draft form. The following format shown in *Box 4.3* is the conventional way the Donabedian standard is set out.

The draft standard should be circulated to teams, wards, departments, the midwifery manager, medical staff and other interested parties for comments. Group members should take the draft standard to changeovers to discuss it with colleagues or other general discussion sessions set up when staff are available. This is a good way of disseminating information and ideas and getting feedback. Other ways are to put suggested standards on a notice board set aside for this purpose. This means that staff on night duty and others who do not get to general discussion groups can give feedback. Cascading information about standards through meetings such as senior staff meetings is also an effective way of giving information, getting feedback and getting people 'on board.' Feedback should be taken seriously and brought back to the group for consideration.

Several redrafts may be necessary before a general consensus is reached. A start date needs to be decided. The standard then needs to be ratified and signed. This is the job of the midwifery manager.

Copies of the finalized standard should be sent to all wards and departments. A standards folder can be made for each area so that all standards, samples of leaflets or other literature connected with standards and

Box 4.3   The conventional way of setting out a Donabedian standard using an example from Nottingham City Hospital

Ward standard no. 1   **Date:** 1st May 1996

City Hospital (NHS Trust) Maternity Unit

Clinical area: Maternity wards

Standard statement: All mothers will be offered privacy during their stay on the ward

STRUCTURE	PROCESS	OUTCOME
All maternity unit staff	Midwife will inform mothers of right to privacy on admission	Mothers will know how to obtain privacy
Single rooms		
Curtains/screens		
'Do not enter' signs	Midwife will demonstrate facilities available	Mothers will feel that their need for privacy is respected
Patient's Charter Standard No. 1 (Department of Health, 1991)		

MONITORING TOOL

Interview mothers every 12 months at postnatal discharge:

1. Do you feel you were offered privacy whilst on the ward? Yes/No
2. Do you feel you could obtain privacy if you wanted it? Yes/No

Midwifery Manager (signature)

subsequent audits can be filed with it. This should be put in an accessible place, so that it can be referred to and students and new staff can familiarize themselves with it.

The next standard

If a group was convened to concentrate on a particular area such as labour suite, antenatal clinic or postnatal care then the group can continue to meet and set standards for that area. If, however, the group was convened to consider a particular specialist subject such as ethnic issues or security the group can be disbanded when the standard has been set and other groups can be formed in the same way from other interested trained volunteers to look at another area that may have emerged as a particular problem or area of concern.

Key points

- The quality co-ordinator sets up quality groups.

- Groups may be set up around clinical areas or specific subjects.

- Group size should be between 6–12 people.

- Meetings should be held every 3–4 weeks, and away from clinical demands.

- Open sharing of ideas is encouraged, hierarchies are discouraged.

(*continued opposite*)

(continued)

- Brainstorming is a useful method for generating creative ideas.

- One standard should be worked on at a time in the group.

- Having set one standard, groups may continue to set others or disband and other group(s) formed.

- All staff should be given opportunities to feedback comments and suggestions and so 'own' the standard for themselves.

References

Clegg F (1990) *Simple Statistics*. Cambridge University Press: Cambridge.

Department of Health (1991) *The Patient's Charter*. HMSO: London.

Department of Health (1993) *The Patient's Charter. Monitoring Made Easy*. HMSO: London. p. 28.

Kirk J and Miller M (1986) *Reliability and Validity in Qualitative Research*. Sage Publications: Newbury Park, California.

Rowntree D (1981) *Statistics without Tears*. Penguin Books Ltd: London.

Wilson CRM (1987) *Hospital-Wide Quality Assurance*. WB Saunders, Toronto. p. 75.

Section *3* Measuring Quality

5 Coordinating Audit

There is little point in setting standards if they are not monitored. They will literally become a paper exercise. Initiatives may be implemented, changes may come about, but if outcomes are not measured it will not be known whether real improvements have been made or are being sustained.

Audits need to be planned. They do not happen on their own. Timing is important. As stated before, it is important to avoid unrepresentative times e.g. bank holidays or weekends, though for a longer audit this may be unavoidable. Audits are time consuming and can produce stress. If possible, periods of time when there are acute staffing problems should be avoided, unless of course the audit concerns staffing levels or other issues associated with staffing.

Audits do not 'run themselves.' Whether carried out frequently or infrequently, a coordinator is always needed to oversee the audit, to give a sense of direction, and to check that it is carried out in the way originally planned when the standard was set and ratified. It is the job of the quality coordinator to coordinate audits or to make sure that a specific person has the responsibility for doing this task.

Preparation

Preparation is the key to the success of audits and falls into two main categories: preparation of people and preparation of materials.

Preparation of People

If staff are expected to take part in audits, they need information, resources and support. It is important that the staff are not only aware that audits are being carried out, but also whether they are expected to take part and exactly how. The quality coordinator needs to be enthusiastic about the audit and willing to explain over and over again its purpose. If she or he is not enthusiastic, it is highly unlikely that anyone else will be either!

There are different ways of communicating this information and ideally all of them should be used. One way of ensuring success is to talk to those who are to be involved so that any questions can be asked. Changeovers or other times when the staff are together are ideal opportunities.

The information should also be taken to senior staff meetings to be 'cascaded' down to team or department members. Posters displayed in strategic places explaining the purpose of the audit and when it will start are a good idea, and should be put up 2–3 weeks ahead of the audit.

Sample questionnaires and interviews should be shown to staff with instructions on how and when to administer them. Staff should be reminded that mothers must be asked whether they are happy to answer questions and told that their answers will be anonymous. Mothers ought to be allowed to decline to take part if they wish with no pressure put on them. If a mother does decline, this should be noted on the questionnaire or interview schedule and collected with the completed ones. To avoid bias, the questions ought to be asked in the same way and mother's actual replies noted. They should not be interpreted and answers must not be suggested.

Preparation of Materials

If the monitoring tool is a questionnaire or an interview schedule they will need to be produced in sufficient numbers. It is important that there are clear instructions for the staff or mothers on the materials with the name of the unit, and details of what the audit is about and what to do with the completed form. Pens or pencils should be supplied for mothers in case they do not have their own. Thanks to those participating in an audit should always be put at the bottom of the form or questionnaire or communicated verbally.

Sufficient supplies of materials need to be available along with a box or large envelope for completed questionnaires or interview schedules.

Making audits as easy as possible for staff to carry out will greatly improve the response rate.

During the audit

The person responsible for coordinating the audit should be available to answer questions at the beginning of the audit and be accessible throughout. It is important that there is an interest in how the audit is going. This will keep people aware of the audit. Clinical needs must always remain the priority, but keeping awareness high will ensure that audits are not forgotten.

There will be some staff who are reluctant to take part in audits. This can sometimes be overcome by trying to find out the reason. It could be the design of the monitoring tool. It may be too time consuming to carry out, or questions may be ambiguous, in which case it needs to be adapted. If staff are very busy with clinical demands audits may, understandably, take low priority. If these issues become a major problem they should be taken back to the standard setting group for resolution. Maintaining adequate supplies of materials is imperative. Audits cannot be carried out without the tools.

When the audit has finished, the staff should be thanked for taking part in person, by posters and in the subsequent audit report.

Key points

- Making audits as easy as possible for staff will increase the response rate.

- Staff should be informed well in advance about the purpose and timing of audits, and shown the material they will be expected to complete.

- Adequate supplies of materials should be prepared, along with instructions about completion.

- The quality coordinator should be easily accessible to answer queries.

---

6 Making Sense of Audit Results

The credibility and value of any results and the subsequent evaluation can only be at the end of a well thought out and executed audit plan.

Once all the data have been collected, what then? How can we make sense of all the data in the vast piles of paper? More importantly, how can we find out what they mean and what the implications are for practice?

Midwives, in common with other health professionals, have traditionally been good at collecting data, but not so good at evaluating them (Walshe and Coles, 1993). They have systematically documented normal delivery and caesarian section rates and postpartum haemorrhage and episiotomy rates. They have not been so good at evaluating the data and asking what these results mean. Are they acceptable or unacceptable? How do they compare with last month, last year, other units or national rates? Rarely have they used the results to look at practice, to change and improve it.

The main aims of examining audit data are as follows given in *Box 6.1.*

Box 6.1 *The main aims of examining audit data*

- To provide an analysis of the results that puts them into context, comparing them with other audit results, where appropriate, and relating them to the standard.

- To present the results in written and verbal form in an unbiased way that makes sense, gives a basis for discussion and subsequent change, and is a source of information for the future.

Analysing data need not be a complicated process. Indeed, many audits produce simple data that are easy to analyse. Although statistical tests can be carried out on audit data, in many audits there are not sufficient numbers. However, this does not necessarily devalue the data (Kirk and Miller, 1986).

The three important questions will be considered separately to ask when looking at audit data are listed in *Box 6.2.*

Box 6.2 *Three important questions when looking at audit data*

- What are the results?

- What do they mean?

- What should be done?

What are the results?

A large part of analysing data consists of counting and categorizing. Counting up data, expressing them as percentages, and putting them into categories forms the basis of many audits. It is important that both numbers and percentages are available. Just presenting numbers on their own may be misleading. For example, finding that 400 mothers were induced last year does not mean much. Was it 400 of 2500 deliveries (16%) or 400 of 5500 deliveries (7.3%)? The answer makes a big difference to subsequent discussion and the conclusions drawn. Percentages should also not be presented on their own. An '80% response rate' sounds impressive. However, if that 80% represents only eight respondents, it is not so impressive!

When starting to look at the data, the first thing to ascertain is how many (as a number and a percentage) of the questionnaires, interviews or other audit tools were completed. This is the response rate. Only rarely will there be a 100% response rate. Some interviews or questionnaires will be forgotten by staff, some would-be respondents will decline, and yet others may be unable to take part because they are not literate or there is a language barrier. If the reasons for non-completion are known this should be indicated in the report. If questionnaires are used, a higher response rate is likely if the mother is prompted or reminded to respond in some way than if she is left to remember to complete and return it herself. It is important to know the response rate when the overall results are considered. The results of an audit with a 10% response rate would be considered very differently from a 90% response rate.

The rest of the data may now be looked at. If it is a questionnaire or interview the answers to the questions should be worked through systematically.

Closed Questions

Answers to closed questions will usually be 'yes/no/don't know,' a tick list or a Likert type scale with pre-determined answers. The simplest way of analysing this kind of data is to count up the yes's, nos and don't knows or other fixed replies and express them as totals and percentages. As the replies are grouped, they can be presented in a table such as *Table 6.1*.

Table 6.1   *Were mothers given an information leaflet about vitamin K?*

Reply	No.	%
Yes	70	85
No	5	6
Don't know	3	4
Not completed	4	5
Total	82	100

Open Questions

Open questions produce data that also need to be categorized. They are more difficult to analyse because their nature is to give respondents an opportunity to answer in their own way without being prompted. This may lead to as many different answers as there are respondents. The best way to deal with these data is to sort them into categories. As the data are examined, several similar types of answer will often emerge. These can be grouped into categories and listed in descending numerical order. For example, in an audit concerning mothers obtaining help with breastfeeding, the question 'Any other comments?' may elicit replies such as 'conflicting advice,' 'good support,' 'not enough help.' The results after the replies have been categorized may look like those shown in *Table 6.2.*

Table 6.2 Comments about help with breastfeeding

Comments	No.	%
Good support	51	61.5
Helpful advice	17	20.5
Not enough help	9	10.8
Conflicting advice	4	4.8
No comment	2	2.4
Total	83	100

In an open question at the end of a questionnaire or interview schedule asking for 'any other comments', there may be many diverse comments and it may be difficult to put them into any sort of category. For example, in a questionnaire in an antenatal clinic there may be complaints about long waiting times, compliments about the helpful and caring staff, and suggestions for more facilities such as better crèche facilities or more magazines. A helpful way of categorizing these responses is into positive comments, negative comments and suggestions. These categories can then be explained and examples of direct quotes given. Again, data in each category should be expressed in both numbers and percentages.

Numerical Data

Some audit results are numerical, for example, lengths of time or blood test results such as haemoglobin concentrations. As with answers to open questions there may be as many different answers as there are respondents. The data therefore need to be sorted into categories. Lengths of time can be grouped into categories such as

0–20 minutes, 21–40 minutes and more than 40 minutes according to the audit being carried out. Sometimes the categories will be obvious and relate to an already existing standard, for example the Patient's Charter standard of outpatients being seen within 30 minutes (Department of Health, 1991).

Data such as postnatal haemoglobin concentrations will also need to be grouped. Again, an obvious category would be an internationally recognized standard such as the World Health Organization (1972) definition of postnatal anaemia as a haemoglobin (Hb) concentration of less than 10 g/dl. Data could be grouped into two categories: haemoglobin concentration over or equal to 10 g/dl and haemoglobin concentration less than 10 g/dl. Other subgroups may also be created. An example is given in *Table 6.3*. If recognized standards are used the results can be compared with those of other studies of the subject.

Table 6.3   *Postnatal haemoglobins 1994*

Haemoglobin	No.	%
> = 10 g/dl	4330	77.7
9–10 g/dl	723	13.0
< 9 g/dl	512	9.2

'Other' Data and Odd Data

In most audits, there will be data which do not appear to be relevant or valid. The questionnaire may been filled in wrongly, the data may not make sense, the answer may not relate to the question, or there may be two answers when only one was asked for.

Some data will be impossible to interpret, e.g. the times entered indicates that the mother was seen for her appointment before she arrived at the clinic! In this sort of case, it is best to discount the data as invalid. Other data that appear irrelevant to a particular question may be included under 'any other comments' data. Data that do not fit easily in any particular category can be put in a category called 'Other' and an explanation given in the text of the report. Whatever happens, the data need to be accounted for.

What do the results mean?

Once the results have been analysed they need to be evaluated. Evaluation has been defined as 'judging the value of something by making a comparison' (Ovretveit, 1992). Another helpful definition is that it is a 'critical assessment, on as objective basis as possible, of the degree to which entire services or their component parts fulfil stated goals (St Leger *et al.*, 1992).

What was the response rate? As mentioned above, results from a 10% response rate should be treated with much more caution than those from a 90% response rate. With a low response rate it is difficult to be sure that the results are representative of the rest of the sample or population. Most audits, however, if carried out properly, will have a response rate of 70% or more, particularly if interviews are the audit tool.

An overview needs to be taken of the main results. Are they acceptable or not? By whose standards? Great care is needed to ensure that discussion and conclusions are as free of bias as possible and that results are not selectively used to make the outcome seem better. Facts do not stand on their own. So-called 'facts' may just be carefully selected statistics. They need to be interpreted, that is, put into context.

Some results will obviously be good results. A 97% rate of satisfaction with care is clearly acceptable. A 3%

rate is not. If this is the first audit, the standard setting group will need to look at the result, decide what is acceptable, and see how far they need to go to meet the standard.

One obvious way of making sense of the results and putting them into context is to compare them with other audits of the same subject. In this way it can be seen whether or not an improvement has taken place. For example, 80% of mothers may have received the advice and help they needed in the present audit. If the previous result was 60% they are subject to a different interpretation than if the previous result was 95%. Over a period of time with several results, it is often possible to see patterns or trends emerging. A good (or bad) result may be a 'one off' or emerge as part of a trend.

Sometimes results from different questions contradict each other. The reason why this has happened needs to be considered. The cause may be ambiguous or confusing questions or the replies may be genuinely contradictory. A respondent may for example indicate that she did not receive a bottle feed demonstration, but then in a further question comment that she found the demonstration helpful! In this case it may be decided to discard the data or report the results as they are with the apparent discrepancies.

Graphs, Bar Charts, Pie Charts

Plotting results on bar charts and pie charts will often give an immediate impression of the results, which cannot be achieved through a simple presentation of tabulated results. *Figure 6.1* shows the data from *Table 6.1* in the form of a pie chart. *Figures 6.2* and *6.3* show the data from *Table 6.2* as both a pie chart and a bar chart. Presenting data in this way makes more impact than presenting data in a table. Where there are small numbers of data however, tables may be more appropriate.

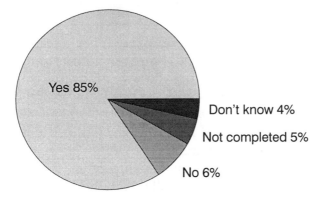

Figure 6.1 *Were mothers given vitamin K information?*

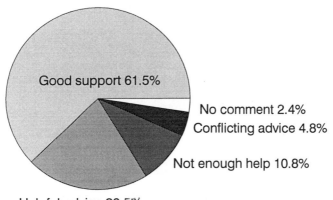

Figure 6.2 *Pie chart illustrating mothers' comments about breastfeeding.*

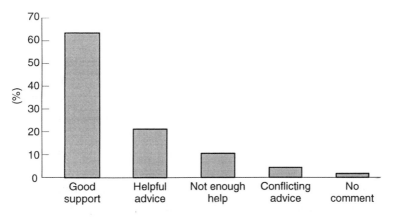

Figure 6.3 *Bar chart illustrating mothers' comments about breastfeeding.*

When other similar audits have been carried out in the unit and like can be compared with like, the results can be plotted on a graph to give an overall impression of trends. *Figure 6.4* shows the results of several monthly audits of the percentages of low postnatal haemoglobins of mothers who had normal deliveries. It can be clearly seen that the overall trend is down.

This consideration and evaluation is the discussion part of the report which will be produced

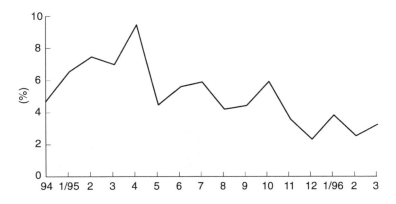

Figure 6.4 *Percentage of women who had a normal delivery and a low postnatal haemoglobin concentration (i.e. less than or equal to 9 g/dl) 1994–1996*

What should be done?

The measurement and evaluation has now been carried out. The issue now is what to do with the results. This is the most important part of the whole process, the *raison d'être* of the audit. Indeed evaluation without action has been called 'an essentially sterile process' (Walshe and Coles, 1993).

Where possible, there should be a discussion of the initial results in the standard setting group. Some changes will be obvious. The quality coordinator will draw conclusions about what needs to change and possibly make some suggestions as to how the change can be implemented as part of the discussion in her or his report. Presenting the findings in a written report is the next important step in this process.

Presenting reports

Results and their evaluation need to be presented in written form. This has the effect of formalizing the results and making them accessible. Results which are not presented will quickly be forgotten. They are useful for reference and for comparison with future audits and as a resource.

Writing reports need not be a prolonged exercise. It is important, however, that reports are written in a way that makes the results accessible, understandable and logical. Tables and figures should be numbered and given a title that describes the contents. The main points that should be covered, however briefly, in an audit report are listed in *Box 6.3*.

Copies of the report need to be sent to group members, the midwifery manager, medical staff where relevant, all wards and departments (to be eventually filed for future reference) and other interested or involved parties.

It is important that the results are taken back to the standard setting group and that it has the opportunity to consider the results and contribute to the discussion before changes are made. This encourages ownership of the results. The results can be discussed at staff meetings, and ward or audit meetings and opportunity given for feedback and suggestions for improving results.

As well as discussing the results informally, if possible audit results should also be presented verbally. This improves dissemination of information and gives

Box 6.3   Writing reports: points that should be covered

- Unit name

- Title and subtitle (e.g. audit of labour suite standard no. I: how long do mothers wait to be sutured?)

- Short introduction (include standard statement)

- Method (how the information was collected, dates)

- Results

- Discussion

- Conclusions, recommendations and actions

- Next audit and acknowledgements

- Name, position and date

---

people a chance to ask questions, give feedback and suggest how standards can be improved. Suitable forums are research interest groups, audit groups, perinatal mortality meetings or meetings set up on an ad hoc basis to present audit results. The more staff involved, the greater the likelihood that subsequent change will happen.

Key points

- Audit data need to be analysed and evaluated to produce information about whether standards are being met.

- Audit results should be presented in written form and if possible verbally.

- Ownership of the results is vital for change to take place.

- An action plan should be produced as a result of the evaluation after staff have had the opportunity to give feedback.

References

Department of Health (1991) *The Patient's Charter*. HMSO: London. p. 14.

Kirk J and Miller M (1986) *Reliability and Validity in Qualitative Research*. Sage Publications: Newbury Park, California.

Ovretveit J (1992) *Health Service Quality. An Introduction to Quality Methods for Health Services*. Blackwell Scientific Publications: Oxford.

St Leger A, Schneiden H and Walsworth–Bell J (1992) *Evaluating Health Services' Effectiveness*. Open University Press: Milton Keynes.

Walshe K and Coles J (1993) *Evaluating Audit. Developing a Framework*. CASPE Research: London. p. 5.

World Health Organization (1972) *Nutritional Anaemias*. Technical Series 503.

Section 4 Improving Quality

7 Implementing Change

'Effective audit may be regarded as a three part cycle of setting standards, evaluating care, and modifying practice in the light of the evaluation. Many audits fail in the last stage because there is no formal feedback of information and no formal decision to remedy the deficiencies that are discovered. Without feedback and remedy "orphan data" merely accumulate' (Shaw, 1980).

'Unless behaviour changes, nothing changes' (Plant, 1987).

There is little point in carrying out audit or, for that matter, setting standards if changes based on the comparison of the reality with the expected outcome are not made. Audits may be performed, and reports can be presented, but unless change takes place they are at best an interesting exercise, at worst a waste of time and resources.

Back in the 1970s, Brook (1977) stated that 'the central failing of quality assessment is that it has rarely been used to change behaviour and hence has not contributed much to the goal of improving the health of the American people.'

More recently in a British context, Walshe and Coles (1992) had this to say about the failure of audit findings to improve care: '... much evaluative research regardless of its conclusions seems to have little or no impact on what happens or how things are done.'

Even when a problem is recognized, changes are not always made (Smith, 1990), and when change is attempted, it can be 'notoriously hard to achieve' (Crombie and Davies, 1992).

These views may be too pessimistic, but there seems to be little question that many good audit or quality assurance programmes have failed to deliver because, for a variety of reasons, changes based on the audit findings were not made. Carrying out audits is an integral part of the quality cycle. However, by themselves they will not effect change no matter how well they are carried out, how accurate the results, or how compelling the conclusions.

In this chapter we will look at first, how and why people change; secondly, the factors that influence people to change their practice; lastly, how these factors can be harnessed to produce lasting change in clinical practice.

Changing midwifery

People and practices change no matter how slowly or imperceptibly. Midwives and midwifery are no exception. Midwifery has gone through tremendous changes since the 1970s. Then, care for women was medically orientated and characterized in pregnancy by frequent visits to 'cattle market' hospital antenatal clinics and in labour by routine shaves and enemas, high induction rates of up to 60% or even 70% (Robinson, 1995), routine amniotomy, the application of fetal scalp electrodes, and in some hospitals, routine intrauterine pressure catheters and episiotomies (Kitzinger, 1979).

After labour, postnatal care was also medically orientated. The discharge examination for all types of delivery was carried out by the obstetrician and mothers who had an instrumental delivery commonly stayed in hospital for a fixed length of time. Four-hourly feeding was the norm, breastfeeds were timed, and breastfed babies were often given complementary feeds. Test weighing was common. Some hospitals had a policy of giving all babies a first feed of water or dextrose by a midwife in case the baby had a tracheo-oesophageal fistula. Serum bilirubins were taken by doctors and it was common practice for babies to be discharged by a paediatrician (in addition to the newborn check) before discharge home.

Times have changed. Care of the pregnant, labouring and delivered mother and her baby has become more midwife orientated, with more emphasis on normality, individualized care and informed choice.

Even before *Changing Childbirth* (Cumberledge Report, 1993), the care of mothers had changed to become more individualized and personalized. Midwives have developed (or regained) their skills, becoming once again the experts in the care of normal pregnancy, labour and puerperium. They are also developing other skills such as intravenous cannulation, caring for mothers having mobile epidurals, transitional care and examination of the newborn. Midwifery practice has therefore undergone tremendous changes.

So people and practice can and do change, but how does it come about and how can positive change be facilitated? Lewin (1951) suggested that change involves a process of unfreezing (become aware of the problem and need to change); moving (being influenced by others to take action); and refreezing (integration of the change).

Rogers (1983) found that people fall into distinct categories. Those who take on change first tend to be 'innovators.' They are risk takers and get their ideas from outside sources, for example, publications in journals and conferences. However, if the change is to be taken on board throughout an organization, 'early adopters' then need to be persuaded of the need for change. They are generally opinion leaders who have influence and are able to persuade the 'early' and 'late majority' to go along with the changes. Lastly there are the 'laggards,' who adopt change in varying degrees, if at all. The uptake of innovations classically follows an 'S' shape (*Figure 7.1*). People respond, then, in different ways to change. This may be partly due to their personality, but will also be influenced by other factors. Early adopters tend to be more educated, of higher social status, more empathetic and less dogmatic than late adopters (Rogers, 1983). The more senior innovators and opinion leaders are, the more likely they are to influence change.

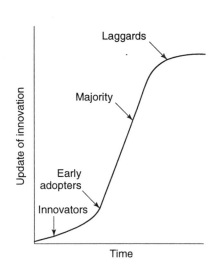

Diffusion

Laggards

Majority

Update of innovation

Early
adopters

Innovators

Time

Figure 7.1 *Diffusion of uptake of innovations (Stocking, 1992). Reproduced with permission from the BMJ Publishing Group*

Influences on midwives

How is change brought about? Midwives, in common with other health professionals, do not practise in a vacuum. They practise not only as individuals, but also in a social context involving mothers and their families, midwifery colleagues and other health professionals, and in a local, national and international context. We shall examine these influences and their relationship to change in midwifery.

Individual Influences

Midwives are individuals with their own sets of beliefs and value systems acquired both inside and outside their work. How they approach change will depend to some extent on these values. Midwives who have practised for a long time may find it hard to come to terms with changing practices simply because of having done something one way for a long time, it may have become part of their value system.

An example of how change in practice may clash with deeply held values and beliefs is serum screening for Down's syndrome. Many midwives have objections to the test on ethical or religious grounds. Although Government policy is that all mothers should be offered the test (Department of Health, 1993), in practice maternity units have varied a great deal in how comprehensively they have taken on the screening with large national differences in the uptake of the test. In some units for example, the test is carried out on an 'opt-in' basis, in others on an 'opt-out' basis, and in others it is not offered at all (Sullivan, 1996). Concern has been expressed in one study that 25% of midwives (who do most of the counselling for the test) were not in favour of the test and 33% did not feel termination of pregnancy for Down's syndrome was justified (Khalid *et al.*,

1994). It is likely that these attitudes and beliefs are a reflection of those held by the people who make the decisions about the implementation of screening tests (i.e. obstetricians, GPs and midwives) and it is therefore likely that this is at least part of the reason for the uneven uptake of the test throughout the country.

While it is unlikely that quality initiatives will raise ethical dilemmas, deeply held beliefs and their subsequent effect on the uptake of change should not be underestimated.

Local Influences

Midwives work in a local environment, be it a hospital unit or a community team. They are influenced by local protocols, policies, standards and the people with whom they work. Their practice involves many other disciplines whose practice impinges on their own and their position in the organization will affect how much they influence or are influenced by others.

Locally produced audits also have the potential of influencing practice. They have the advantage of being carried out in a local context and do not therefore have the remoteness of audits or research that have been carried out elsewhere. The results are therefore easier to own. However, it is important that local audit results and subsequent recommendations are seen to be produced from a credible source and not by managers or administrators whose motives may be mistrusted or expertise may be doubted (Robertson *et al.*, 1996).

Consumers' views may also influence practice (Bark *et al.*, 1994). The situation has changed a great deal since the 1970s when the statement could be made that 'the consumer is in no way able to make judgements about the clinical care he gets' (Klein, 1973). Consumer satisfaction surveys, *The Patient's Charter* (Department of Health, 1991) and the policies of individual units make complaining easier and as a result the number of complaints has risen dramatically over the last few years, up to fivefold (Bark *et al.*, 1994). This does not necessarily reflect that the service is worse, just that consumers are more aware of their rights and complaining has been made easier. Even 'questioning or demanding patients' can affect practice (Stocking, 1992).

External Influences

External forces affect midwives in many ways. Midwives' practice is regulated by the United Kingdom Central Council for Nursing, Midwifery and Health Visiting, *The Midwives' Code of Practice* (1994) and *Midwives' Rules* (1993) and by statute.

Publications issued by the Department of Health reflecting government policy, for example *The Patient's Charter* (1991), *The Maternity Charter* (1994) and *Changing Childbirth* (Cumberledge Report, 1993) have had a great influence on midwifery practice as does practice in other units such as that reported in midwifery and medical journals and at national and international conferences.

Midwives' practice is also influenced by lay organizations such as the National Childbirth Trust (NCT) and Association for Improvements in Maternity Services (AIMS), and by public opinion expressed through the media.

Sometimes several of these forces combine, either locally or in the wider context, adopting an impetus of their own to produce a 'climate of opinion' (Stocking, 1992). The changing of the law in 1996 regarding the handcuffing of women prisoners in labour is one such example. Consumer groups, politicians and the Royal College of Midwives combined to put pressure on the government to change the law.

Some years ago, the care of mothers who had a stillbirth was very different to what is accepted today.

Several factors were responsible for this, not least the effect of public opinion. Good professional practice has developed so that the care of mothers and their families after the loss of a baby is more sensitive and supportive. A return to the days when a stillborn baby was taken away from the mother without her being given the chance or choice to see her baby is almost inconceivable.

The 'climate of opinion,' however, is not always a force for good. After an influential lecture in the Netherlands in the 1970s, medical opinion and the media created a climate of opinion that recommended that babies sleep prone rather than supine in the belief, along with other reasons, that babies could breathe better (Engleberts and DeJonge, 1990). This unfortunately proved to be a disaster as there was a subsequent rise in cot death rates (Engleberts and DeJonge, 1990). It was only in the late 1980s that this practice was questioned leading to a subsequent change in the climate of opinion that babies should sleep in the supine position and a dramatic fall of 40% in the cot death rate in 1988 compared with that of 1987 (Engleberts and DeJonge, 1990).

Midwives are influenced by research. The publication of research by Romney (1980) and Romney and Gordon (1981) showing that routine shaves and enemas in labour were at best ineffectual and at worst harmful had a great influence on midwifery practice. As a result, these procedures became outdated and are no longer part of routine midwifery practice.

However, research does not always change practice. Many practices have been carried out for years and people may see no good reason to change, even if the proposed change is research based (Stocking, 1992). Swabbing the perineum in labour, for example, is a well established practice that has been perceived to be beneficial to the mother in reducing the danger of infection, as well as being a 'comfort' procedure. Even if research indicated that there are no benefits, the feeling that it is right to carry out swabbing may be so ingrained that it could take a long time to overcome the practice. Staff need to be convinced that the benefits of not carrying out, changing or instituting a new procedure outweigh the major psychological hurdles of overcoming individual beliefs to change a long established practice.

Even some simple changes can be difficult to implement or alternatively having made them, people may slip back into their old habits. It has been suggested that complex change is easier to implement than simple change (Stocking, 1992) because people have to compromise and adapt with more complicated change, and 'there is no going back.' Simple change may not continue if the initiator of the change moves on.

The impetus for change therefore comes from many different directions. But this does not make change inevitable. People need to be convinced not only that the change is advantageous, but that it will work and that all objections have been thought through and dealt with (Stocking, 1992).

If people are influenced by their value systems and philosophies, opinion leaders, research and audit findings, and the general climate of opinion, it is clear that great attention should be paid to communication. People need to have access to ideas, research and audit results. However, as already discussed, results on their own will not effect change. As we have seen, people want to change in different ways and the implementation of change needs to take this into account. Results and suggestions should be presented in a way that makes sense, that is broadly in line with people's values and philosophies, and makes people feel as though they have a say. Ownership is vital if midwives are to implement change.

Successful change

Successful change results from managing people well

and using methods that help people through the process of change. Good communication is at the heart of successful change.

People

Introducing change does not mean dismantling the whole system (Ovretveit, 1992). It means building on what is already there. It is often better to adapt than adopt.

People, depending to some extent on their position in the organization, personalities and other factors will have varying propensities and abilities to take on and implement change. 'Innovators' and 'early adopters' will be influenced by external sources such as research and conferences. Early adopters tend to be 'opinion leaders' who influence the 'majority,' and are the key to successful change in the organization (Rogers, 1983). Great attention therefore needs to be paid to the way change is communicated in the organization.

In their 'checklist for good audit', Crombie and Davies (1992) listed: a planned programme in which all staff were involved, active feedback and a further evaluation of changes. Before change can be implemented there needs to be agreement about what the underlying problems or needs are and consensus about what to do, how and when (Crombie and Davies, 1993). To do this there needs to be active feedback (Crombie and Davies, 1992; Robertson *et al.*, 1996). This consists of giving all staff an opportunity to comment and contribute to the discussion about what is the problem, what needs to be done, who is to be involved and when. It is important to communicate results to and get feedback from as wide an audience as possible in different ways and as soon as possible (Mugford *et al.*, 1991). This should include those who are 'on the shop floor' as well as managers. A simple dissemination of results alone will not achieve change (Stocking, 1992)

Managers need to be involved throughout the planning process to support the change and so that change can be resourced. Indeed encouragement from all senior staff is helpful in implementing change (Mansfield, 1995).

A plan needs to be produced setting out timescales and what has been agreed. This has the function of focusing the change, keeping awareness high, and giving authority to the changes.

Methods

Good communication is at the heart of successful change. Great attention therefore needs to be paid to the methods of implementing change. If they are to work, they should include all staff, be accessible and easy to understand. They will be those methods that facilitate staff to take on the change.

Education may be needed for certain kinds of change (Mugford *et al.*, 1991; Stocking, 1992; Robertson *et al.*, 1996). This may take the form of lectures or seminars, or if it is a practical skill, practical teaching or demonstration sessions where people can develop their skills.

An effective way of implementing change is to produce guidelines (Stocking, 1992; Mansfield, 1995; Shaw, 1989). These should be 'owned' by those who are expected to follow them (Dukes and Stewart, 1993) and be evidence based (Stocking, 1992; Grol, 1993), but also easy to understand, related to everyday (local) practice, and allowing for clinical judgement or patient preference where appropriate.

Keeping awareness high by giving feedback and regular progress reports will keep people involved and interested. Passive or negative feedback of results or giving clinicians evidence of poor performance alone have been found to be ineffective or even counterproductive, increasing denial of the need to change.

'Trials' are sometimes a good way of introducing change, particularly if people are doubtful about the proposed benefits of change. In this way, it is not necessarily permanent and there is a way back or a way forward without loss of face (Stocking, 1992).

Robertson *et al.* (1996) suggest that trying out several strategies may be more helpful than a single strategy to overcome obstacles to change. However, they warn that this 'scattergun' approach can be impractical and ineffective if indiscriminately used. It is suggested that the likely obstacles to change are identified so that strategies can be tailored to overcome them.

Audits are simply a means to an end. The results need to be owned and acted upon. There needs to be management support to facilitate change and provide motivation, resources and time. It is the job of the quality coordinator to make sure that the work is taken forward and does not lose impetus.

The strategies for successful change are listed in *Box 7.1*.

Box 7.1   Strategies for change that work

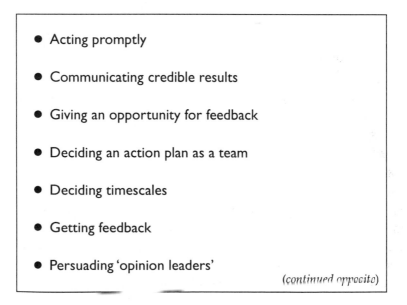

- Acting promptly

- Communicating credible results

- Giving an opportunity for feedback

- Deciding an action plan as a team

- Deciding timescales

- Getting feedback

- Persuading 'opinion leaders'

(continued opposite)

(*continued*)

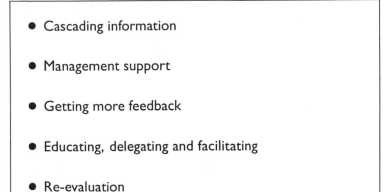

- Cascading information

- Management support

- Getting more feedback

- Educating, delegating and facilitating

- Re-evaluation

Managing change

'Change comes from small initiatives which work which, imitated, become the fashion. We cannot wait for great visions from great people. We must light our own small fires in the darkness.' (Charles Handy, quoted in Royal College of Speech and Language Therapists, 1996)

In view of the foregoing discussion, it can be seen that some strategies work better than others in effecting change. How then can change be implemented successfully on the 'shop floor'?

It should be clear by now that communication plays a large part in this process. Recognizing that people have different positions in the organization and fall into different categories in relation to taking on change is an important first step. Results should be presented in a meaningful and accessible way that encourages feedback and input as to how changes can be made. Results should be taken back to the quality groups, audit meetings and senior staff meetings and an opportunity provided for feedback and suggestions. It may be difficult, if not impossible, to actively involve all staff in discussion. Some may not want to contribute, others may not be easily available. An opportunity for written comments should always be given so that all staff will at least have had the chance to contribute.

It is important that there is a consensus that change is needed, about what needs to be done and who is going to do it. An action plan needs to be agreed by the key people involved in the project, audit or quality group so that all those involved know what is expected of them. Timescales should be planned for the changes and a start date set. This gives time for the information to filter through and to focus the change. The 'opinion leaders' need to be involved in the development of guidelines for better practice and education. This can take the form of posters, leaflets or other easily accessible or visible information, and may be displayed in ward or department areas and staff rooms and on general notice boards. Another way to communicate guidelines is to incorporate them on computer (Mugford *et al.*, 1991). Computer software can be adapted to include prompts to clinicians to carry out tasks or give advice. Flowcharts may also be a good way of communicating new ideas in an accessible form (Grol, 1993; Mansfield, 1995).

At the start date, it is important that the quality coordinator or other designated person checks that the change has indeed started. Time needs to be given for change to take root. It has been suggested that it takes three times as much time for guidelines to be implemented as for their design (Dukes and Stewart, 1993). It seems sensible to assume that the principle holds no matter how the change is planned and effected.

After the change has been introduced it is vital that a re-evaluation takes place to ensure that the change has in fact occurred. As Smith (1990) said 'Without this "closing of the feedback loop," audit may be little more than a pious exercise in self congratulation.'

Unsuccessful change

Walshe and Coles (1993) attribute failure to change to 'poor dissemination, a lack of incentives to change, an unwillingness to accept unwelcome results, a lack of credibility on the part of the evaluation itself, a tendency to discover that the evaluation posed (and answered) the wrong questions....' If good communication is at the heart of successful change, then poor communication will be a main cause of failure to implement change.

People

Reasons why people fail to change have been accounted for from several different perspectives (Robertson *et al.* 1996). It may be explained at a personal level: perhaps the clinician lacks the skills or confidence to make the change. An effective strategy in this case is to provide education, positive feedback and guidelines in which clinicians have had input or which come from a credible and respected source.

Failure to implement change may be explained at a group level (i.e. the leaders may be afraid that they will lose power as a result of the changes or clinicians may presume that other colleagues will implement change even though no-one may have been given the specific responsibility). Another reason may be a subgroup resisting change and influencing others to do so as well. A cohesive group which has a strong leadership and belief that the group does not need to change and where dissent is discouraged, will be very hard to influence. Respected outsiders may be able to influence the leaders, and making group members accountable for change may be a successful strategy.

Failure to implement change may also be explained at an organizational level. Clinicians do not effect change because they may feel that outside agents do not have the right to dictate changes (e.g. imposed changes by administration). The option here is to impose change by edict or preferably to improve communication between the opposing groups.

There are other reasons why change may not occur. The changes may challenge deeply held beliefs or long-held practices which people may not be willing to compromise. People may view the suggested changes as impositions and therefore resist them. This may happen as a result of inadequate consultation or feedback. It may, however, reflect the view of people who believe that the change is unworkable. The innovators suggesting the changes need to have either considerable influence themselves or close access to those who do to have any impact on this situation.

Methods

Some methods are unlikely to work and are listed in *Box 7.2*. Disseminating information without explanation and expecting people to change (i.e. passive feedback) is unlikely to work (Mitchell and Fowkes, 1985). Applying research without local adaptation may also fail (Stocking, 1992). Research may sometimes be seen as irrelevant to the local situation and other national audits, opinions or edicts may be seen as being imposed and will therefore be resisted.

Data presented by those outside the unit are unlikely to be trusted (Mugford *et al.*, 1991), and the same applies to routinely obtained data (Crombie and Davies, 1992). People may view the proposed change as 'being invited to accept a procedure which is not founded on science but on a consensus, which may be the views of a majority, the most vociferous, the most influential or the most determined of the designing group' (Dukes and Stewart, 1993).

It is self evident that little or poor planning, support and resourcing will predispose to failure, as will lack of communication or feedback.

Box 7.2   Strategies that do not work

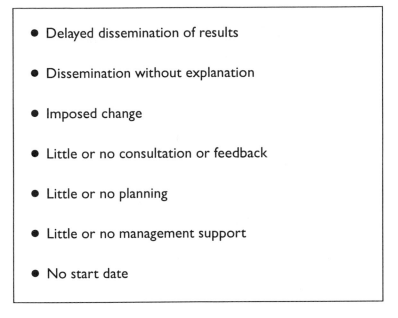

- Delayed dissemination of results

- Dissemination without explanation

- Imposed change

- Little or no consultation or feedback

- Little or no planning

- Little or no management support

- No start date

Conclusion

'Cultures are not changed through contracts, circulars, discussion with august bodies and legislation. Cultures if they are changed are only changed through outstanding leadership and through engaging with every member of the culture. Cultures are not changed from the top but from the bottom, and the art of leadership is to motivate people to want to do what needs to be done.' (Smith, 1995).

People are most likely to change because they want to, not because they have to. Change, if it occurs, will be achieved by clinicians deciding to change and being supported, facilitated and encouraged by their managers and peers. Only then will the quality circle be completed, leading to improved care for mothers and their babies given by midwives and their colleagues, who are constantly evaluating and improving their practice to deliver quality care.

Key points

- There is little point in carrying out audits if the results are not acted upon.

- Change does not happen automatically.

- Good communication is at the heart of successful change.

- Involve everybody as much as possible in the identification of the problem and what to do about it.

- If possible 'adapt rather than adopt.'

- Plan the change and set a start date for the change.

- Educate, delegate and facilitate.

- Implementing change is a vital part of the quality cycle, the so-called 'missing link'.

References

Burk P, Vincent C, Jones A and Savory J (1994) Clinical complaints: a means of improving quality of care. *Quality in Health Care* 3(3): p. 123.

Brook R (1977) Quality – can we measure it? *New England Journal of Medicine* Jan 20: 170–172.

Crombie I and Davies H (1992) Towards good audit. *British Journal of Hospital Medicine* **48** (3): p. 182.

Crombie I and Davies H (1993) Missing link in the audit cycle. *Quality in Health Care* 2: p. 47–48.

Cumberledge Report (1993) *Changing Childbirth. The Report of the Expert Maternity Group.* HMSO. London.

Department of Health (1991) *The Patient's Charter.* HMSO: London.

Department of Health (1994) *The Patient's Charter - Maternity Services.* HMSO: London.

Dukes J and Stewart R (1993) At the cutting edge. *Health Service Journal* **22** April: p 23.

Engleberts A and DeJonge G (1990) Choice of sleeping position for infants: possible association with cot death. *Archives of Disease of Childhood* **65**: 464–467.

Grol R (1993) Development of guidelines for general practice. *British Journal of General Practice* **43**: 146–151.

Khalid L, Price S and Barrow M (1994) The attitudes of midwives to maternal serum screening for Down's syndrome. *Public Health* **108**(2): 131–136.

Kitzinger S (1979) *The Good Birth Guide.* Fontana: Glasgow. pp. 438–439.

Klein R (1973) Who is the patient's friend? *British Medical Journal* 2nd June: 528–532.

Lewin K (1951) *Field Theory in Social Science.* Harper and Row: New York.

Mansfield C (1995) Attitudes and behaviours towards clinical guidelines: the clinician's perspective. *Quality in Health Care* **4**: 250–255.

Mitchell M and Fowkes F (1985) Audit reviewed: Does feedback change clinical behaviour? *Journal of the Royal College of Physicians of London* **19**(4): p. 251.

Mugford M, Banfield P and O'Hanlon M (1991) Effects of feedback of information on clinical practice: a review. *British Medical Journal* **303**: 398–402.

Ovretveit J (1992) *Health Service Quality. An Introduction to Quality Methods for Health Services.* Blackwell Scientific Publications: Oxford. p. 153.

Plant R (1987) *Managing Change and Making it Stick.* Fontana: London.

Robertson N, Baker R and Hearnshaw H (1996) Changing the clinical behaviour of doctors. *Quality in Health Care* **5**: 51–54.

Robinson J (1995) Why mothers fought obstetricians. *British Journal of Midwifery* **3**(10): 557–558.

Rogers EM (1983) *Diffusions of Innovations.* 3rd edn. Free Press: New York. pp. 247–252.

Romney M (1980) Predelivery shaving: an unjustified assault? *Journal of Obstetrics and Gynaecology* **1**: 33–35.

Romney M and Gordon H (1981) Is your enema really necessary? *British Medical Journal* **282**: 1269–1271.

Royal College of Speech and Language Therapists (1996) *Communicating Quality 2: Professional Standards for Speech and Language Therapists.* RCSLT: London.

Shaw C. (1980) Acceptability of audit. *British Medical Journal* 14th June: 1443–1446.

Shaw C (1989) Medical Audit. *A Hospital Handbook.* King's Fund Centre: London. p. 13.

Smith R (1995) Editorial. *British Medical Journal* 12th May: p 402.

Smith T (1990) Medical audit: closing the feedback loop is essential. *British Medical Journal* **300**: 65.

Stocking B (1992) Promoting change in clinical care. *Quality in Health Care* **1**: 56–60.

Sullivan A (1996) Scrum screening for Down's syndrome: the need for knowledge. *British Journal of Midwifery* **4**(4): 183–186.

United Kingdom Central Council for Nursing, Midwifery and Health Visiting (1994) *The Midwives' Code of Practice*. UKCC: London.

United Kingdom Central Council for Nursing, Midwifery and Health Visiting (1993) *Midwives' Rules*. UKCC: London.

Walshe K and Coles J (1993) *Evaluating Audit: Developing a Framework*. CASPE Research: London. p. 6.

8 Examples of Quality

'It must never be lost sight of what observation is for. It is not for the sake of piling up miscellaneous information or curious facts, but for the sake of saving life and increasing health and comfort' (Florence Nightingale, 1875).

This chapter contain real examples of quality initiatives, standards and audit results from Nottingham City Hospital Maternity Unit. Many of the examples are related specifically to antenatal, intrapartum and postnatal care. Others cover broader standards, *The Patient's Charter* (Department of Health, 1991a), professional issues and other quality initiatives.

Much midwifery care is concerned with the amount and quality of information given to mothers to enable them to understand issues related to pregnancy and childbirth and to make informed choices and decisions. The following examples demonstrate this. Over two-thirds of the standards we have set in the Nottingham

City Hospital Maternity Unit are concerned with information giving. Some of the standards were set several years ago when we were just starting to look at quality issues, and the standard statements sometimes reflect this. Nevertheless, the principles remain relevant and may be useful for application in other units, perhaps with modifications.

Antenatal care

Information about Blood Tests

An early standard we set for antenatal mothers concerned information about blood tests offered and carried out. It was set by the Antenatal Clinic Standard Setting Group as 'All women having blood investigations initiated in clinic will understand the reason for the investigation being carried out and will give verbal consent.' All staff, including auxiliary staff, were reminded of the importance of giving explanations for all blood tests and making sure the mother understood and agreed to the test(s). At this time, an attractive poster was designed as part of a course by one of our midwives called '*What, More Blood*?!' explaining simply what the most common antenatal blood tests are carried out for. This was professionally produced by the hospital audiovisual department and is displayed in our clinic outside the phlebotomist's room.

The standard was to be monitored by asking mothers whether they had any blood tests, what they were and whether they had been given an explanation for the tests. Deciding when to ask mothers was difficult. Was the best time just after they had been told about the test, at a later point in the visit, or on the way out of clinic? Asking mothers questions during the clinic visit could have been intrusive. On the way out after the visit was thought to be the best and most practical time. Mothers would be easy to waylay and mothers who were uncertain or had questions could always be referred back or could have the test explained by the interviewing midwife. The tests the mother said she had carried out were checked in her co-operation card.

Midwives from the Standard Setting Group and from clinic agreed to help with the audit and each clinic was monitored for one week. Further audits have been carried out of this standard. *Figure 8.1* shows the results of three audits. As can be seen, over a period of two years there was an improvement both in the percentage of mothers being given an explanation and also in those understanding it.

There were differences between booking and follow-up clinics and these were consistent in all the audits. Mothers who attended for booking clinic seemed more likely to remember being given an explanation for a blood test. It may be that explanations were not always consistently given for 'routine' blood tests such as haemoglobin concentration at follow-up visits. Another explanation could be that mothers generally have more tests at booking clinics and may be more receptive to explanations at that first visit.

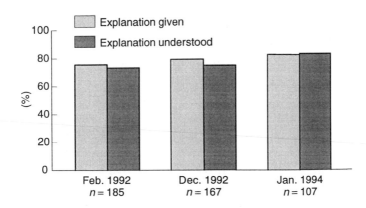

Figure 8.1   *Blood test explanations in antenatal clinic.*

What was interesting was that mothers attending their booking visit were occasionally overheard by the midwife who booked them saying that they had not been given an explanation when they had in fact had been given one! Obviously there are other factors involved. Booking visits may be several hours long and the mother may then forget that she had been given an adequate explanation. Blood tests may not have remained an important issue in the mother's mind once an explanation had been given and the blood had been taken. However, it is clearly important that mothers are given an explanation, particularly for tests for spina bifida and serum screening for Down's syndrome as these tests raise serious ethical issues (Smith *et al.*, 1994).

Their audit also highlighted the fact that mothers whose first language is not English do not always understand the reason for the blood test. This emphasized the need to ask for the help of an interpreter.

Information about Amniocentesis

Amniocentesis is an invasive procedure carried out on a small but significant percentage of mothers. The subject of amniocentesis is often discussed at booking on account of maternal age. It may be raised later on in the pregnancy as a result of abnormal alphafetoprotein or Down's screening test results. It is important that mothers receive accurate information not only about the reason for the test, but also about what is involved, any side effects and when the mother is likely to get the result.

We decided to set a standard about giving information to mothers about amniocentesis. The standard statement stated that 'All women having amniocentesis will understand the reason for the test and what the procedure entails.'

A leaflet was designed by the group after writing to other units and looking at the information in other leaflets. One member of the group wrote the draft, which was commented on by the rest of the group and offered for comments by midwives and obstetricians. We typed and produced it 'in-house.' It contains information about how the procedure is carried out, possible side effects, how long results take to be returned, and a contact number.

Our monitoring tool was incorporated into the leaflet. Two questions were asked: whether the mother understood the reason for amniocentesis; whether she had found the leaflet useful? Space was also left for comments. Mothers were asked to bring the completed questionnaire back to clinic. Community midwives were given copies of the leaflet to give out.

After one year, a study of all the returned questionnaires was carried out. The return rate was disappointingly low at 18%. The reason may have been that many mothers forgot to bring the form back or may not have visited the clinic again in the pregnancy. However, the results were good. All mothers had been given an explanation of the test and all had found the leaflet useful. There were many positive comments both about the leaflet and the staff who carried out or helped with the procedure. Minor amendments to the leaflet were made as a result of some comments.

Waiting Times and Explanations

The Patient's Charter was published by the Department of Health in 1991. Standard no. 6 states that 'Patients will be seen within 30 min of their appointment time.' As all hospitals are required to monitor this standard regularly, we set a similar standard, but added that 'Mothers arriving late will be seen if possible within 30 minutes of their arrival time.'

Many issues influence the amount of time women wait in antenatal clinics. We at the Nottingham City

Hospital Maternity Unit, along with other maternity units in Trent Region looked at the issues in the 1980s (Buckley, 1991a; Buckley, 1991b). Spacing of appointment times and availability of midwifery, obstetric and ultrasonography staff were some of the issues. We made changes to the appointment system to make more effective use of midwifery and ultrasonography staff. Doctors, and in particular, consultants, were asked to attend clinics punctually.

The standard is audited by questionnaire. Mothers are given a form to complete on arrival at the clinic reception desk. They are asked to note down the time 'first seen' by the doctor, midwife or ultrasonographer. Different forms (and different colours for ease of analysis) are given according to whether the visit is a booking, follow-up or scan only.

Figure 8.2 shows the results of audits of waiting times. Between the eight and ninth audits there had been a move to a new maternity unit. This also coincided with a policy change of mothers having extra scans carried out for fetal abnormality at around 18 weeks, which has caused delays.

In addition, the Nottingham City Hospital set a trust standard that 'patients who wait more than 30 minutes to be seen will be given an explanation.' Explanation

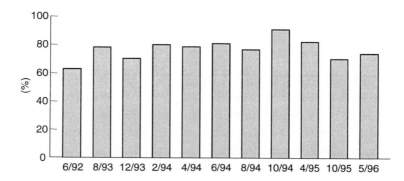

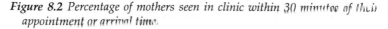

Figure 8.2 *Percentage of mothers seen in clinic within 30 minutes of their appointment or arrival time.*

giving about delays is difficult to institute and monitor. Who should give the explanation and how? How can it be known who has been delayed more than 30 minutes? How can delays be explained? The reasons may vary from the doctor being late because he or she never turns up on time, to the situation where a mother has to be informed that her baby has a congenital abnormality and has to be made aware of the options available to her. To give either reason to a clinic full of waiting mothers would be unacceptable. We decided that it was important that delays were acknowledged with a general explanation such as 'the doctor has been delayed' or 'there is a shortage of staff' and an apology given for the delay.

Auditing the standard was done by asking the question on the same audit form 'If you waited more than 30 minutes to be seen, were you given an explanation for the delay?'

The results of the audit of whether explanations were given has been disappointing. Between 25–37% said they had been given an explanation. This is in spite of the fact that those running the clinic made a lot of effort to ensure mothers did get an explanation and an apology. It may be that the explanations are not perceived as such, or are simply forgotten and therefore not recorded.

Another way of monitoring the standard would be for staff to record when an explanation has been given. However, the same problem of mothers not perceiving what is given as an explanation may still arise. The standard is an example of one which is both difficult to implement and monitor.

Advice about Smoking

The association of smoking with problems in pregnancy is well established (Whent, 1994). It is also recognized that midwives, along with obstetricians, are well placed to warn about the dangers of smoking and give advice and literature to encourage mothers to give up smoking.

The booking visit, be it in the home or in hospital is an ideal time to do this. Mothers are usually early on in their pregnancies and advice and information can be given. However, although this is an important subject, there are of course other competing matters in the booking interview such as obtaining an accurate obstetric and medical history, advice about diet in pregnancy and information about blood tests. Smoking is just one of many important subjects to discuss at the booking interview.

The Antenatal Clinic Standard Setting Group wanted to address the issue, particularly in the light of *The Health of the Nation* (Department of Health, 1992) target that '... at least a third of women smokers to stop smoking at the start of their pregnancy by the year 2000.' At the time, smoking data collected at booking interview consisted of asking the mother whether she smoked and if so, how many cigarettes per day.

Around this time, the District had financed training for every midwife in the hospital and community to give advice to mothers about smoking and pregnancy. As awareness was high, we felt that this was the ideal time to capitalize on heightened awareness. We set a standard stating that 'All mothers who smoke will be given appropriate advice and literature to encourage them to stop smoking.' To implement this standard, we felt that the booking interview was the ideal starting place, but we had to recognize several issues: the need to obtain other important information as mentioned above, the obligation to acquire quantitative data to fulfil contractual obligations and to ascertain whether we were achieving *The Health of the Nation* target, limited time as booking clinics are under constant pressure of time, and the need to have a standardized approach and for it to be 'user-friendly'.

To achieve the standard, we designed an interactive

computer program, incorporated into the existing computer booking interview which produced questions that generated other questions depending on the answers, according to where the mother was on the 'cycle of stopping smoking' (Prochaska and DiClemente, 1983). The program prompts the midwife to ask questions to find out whether the mother and anybody else in the household smokes and if she or they would be willing to give up. Depending on the reply the computer program suggests advice to be given and appropriate leaflets. For example if the mother smokes, the midwife is prompted to give advice about the risks of smoking, the benefits of stopping and how smoking will affect the baby. Whether the mother smokes or not, prompts appear on the screen to remind the midwife to advise all mothers about the dangers of passive smoking. There is a folder containing leaflets that is kept stocked up and easily accessible in each booking room.

All mothers are given the best chance of receiving advice and relevant leaflets wherever she is on the 'cycle of stopping smoking.' She can then be referred to her community midwife for further support or given the 'Quitline' number to get further support and literature.

We have improved the system as a result of staff feedback and amended the suggested leaflets as newer ones have been produced. Nottingham City Hospital was involved in producing the first leaflet in England aimed at partners and families of mothers who smoke and this is used as one of the suggested leaflets for partners. This leaflet is at present being evaluated.

There have been many attempts to influence mothers to give up smoking during pregnancy, some more successful than others (Whent, 1994). In many cases, the problem has been a lack of time or resources or an ad hoc approach with only the 'enthusiasts' giving advice and help. Although the ideal system would allow unlimited time with follow-up support from the same person, time and resource limitations prevent this. We believe we have a pragmatic system that capitalizes on what is already there, facilitates standardized advice giving, and by only suggesting appropriate questions allows effective use of time for targeting information and literature, as recommended by Silargy *et al.* (1996).

The system is in the process of being audited. Information about how many cigarettes the mother smokes the day before delivery is routinely obtained and this is linked with information obtained at booking to evaluate how many mothers give up smoking during pregnancy.

Written Information

Another standard we set for the antenatal clinic involved standardizing the written information given out at booking and making other leaflets, including those in other languages, accessible in clinic.

Intrapartum care

Waiting for Suturing

It is generally acknowledged that there is morbidity subsequent to episiotomy or vaginal or perineal lacerations following delivery. Among these are bleeding (Sleep *et al.* 1989), pain (Howie, 1995), infection (Bennett and Brown, 1989) and haematoma formation (Bobak and Jensen, 1989). Little work, however, appears to have been done on the optimum time to suture, although it has been suggested that prompt suturing secures haemostasis (Bennett and Brown, 1989), promotes healing, limits residual damage and decreases the possibility of infection (Bobak and Jensen, 1989). It is also kinder to the mother (Bennett and Brown, 1989).

Delays in suturing mothers were a cause of verbal and written complaints in our unit. In view of this and the likelihood that there were advantages to suturing mothers promptly, the Labour Suite Standard Setting Group decided to tackle the problem of long delays for perineal suturing after normal delivery as its first standard. It was decided to audit the situation first. Midwives were asked to note down the time of delivery, time of start of perineal suturing, and whether the operator was a midwife or doctor. We found that 44% of mothers waited more than one hour to be sutured, the longest time being 3 hours 12 minutes. Fifty-four percent of mothers were sutured by midwives, 46% by doctors.

The Standard Setting Group decided that an acceptable length of time to wait for suturing was an hour or less. The subsequent standard statement was 'Every mother requiring suturing will be attended to within one hour of delivery.' After multidisciplinary discussion, it was decided that to implement the standard more midwives needed to be trained to suture, and that perineal suturing should take higher priority than other tasks, for instance writing up casenotes. Materials for midwives to practise on were provided as well as other training resources, such as videos.

The time of the start of perineal suturing was entered on computer so that audits could be carried out from computer data. The standard was audited two months later and showed an improvement. With continued monitoring of the standard, it was suggested that some delays were 'avoidable' (e.g. the midwife or doctor being unavailable to suture) and some delays were 'unavoidable' (e.g. maternal or neonatal complications or maternal request). We amended the standard adding the phrase 'unless there are maternal or neonatal complications or maternal request to delay suturing.' We also designed a short questionnaire to appear on computer during the input of delivery data when there had been a delay of more than one hour (*Figure 8.3*).

LABOUR SUITE STANDARD SETTING AUDIT
STANDARD NUMBER 1

This mother waited more than 1 hour to be sutured.

Was the delay due to:

- Maternal condition Y/N   ......

- Baby's condition Y/N   ......

- Maternal request Y/N   ......

- Midwife not available Y/N   ......

- Doctor not available Y/N   ......

Thank you for completing this questionnaire

Figure 8.3 *Computer questionnaire for Labour Suite Standard Setting Audit. Standard number 1.*

After the standard had been amended the 'unavoidable' delays were included in the figures of those sutured in less than one hour. The standard was audited two-monthly, six-monthly and then annually. The results are shown in *Figure 8.4*. The percentage of mothers delayed for more than one hour or avoidably delayed has been reduced from 44% in 1991 to 15% in 1995, a reduction of 65.9%. In 1991, 56% were sutured by

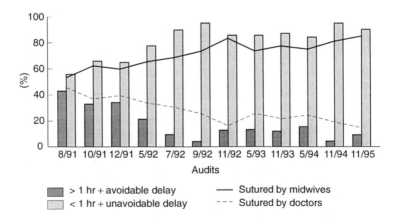

> 1 hr + avoidable delay   —— Sutured by midwives
< 1 hr + unavoidable delay   --- Sutured by doctors

Figure 8.4 *Suturing times after normal delivery.*

midwives whereas in 1995 85% were sutured by mid-wives, an increase of 51.8%.

It seems likely that the reduction in perineal suturing delays is due to the fact that more midwives suture. Since the standard has been implemented, there have been no written complaints about suturing delays. Perineal suturing by midwives is an obvious extension of their role and has the added advantage of giving more continuity of care to mothers.

Waiting for Induction

Waiting for routine induction was the subject of another standard. The Standard Setting Group felt that there was a problem with mothers being admitted for routine induction and having to wait long periods of time to be induced. Mothers were asked to come to the labour suite at 8 a.m. and were sometimes waiting two or three hours until they were seen on the doctors' round and induced. Sometimes mothers were admitted for induction, but because the labour suite was busy, sometimes had to wait for several hours in the sitting room or were sent up the ward to wait. This was considered to be unsatisfactory and stressful for mothers.

It was decided to carry out an audit to see if there was in fact a problem. It was found that 66% of mothers waited more than one hour, some waiting over three hours. A standard was set that stated 'All mothers admitted for routine induction to labour suite will be induced within one hour of the given time of arrival.'

After discussion, it was decided to change the admission time from 8 a.m. to 8.30 a.m. as doctors' rounds rarely started on time, and to produce a leaflet to give to mothers on booking induction. The leaflet is a simple information sheet which fits inside the cooperation card. It records the induction date and asks the mother to ring the labour suite on the morning of induction to check the time of admission. If the labour suite is busy, the mother can be asked to wait at home and come in later.

Figure 8.5 shows the results of audits carried out, the first one being before the standard was set and implemented. As can be seen there is a distinct improvement.

It was also decided to find out the reasons for any delay in induction. A short questionnaire was designed to appear automatically on the computer screen if there was a delay of more than one hour between admission and induction. The possible reasons were 'mother arrived early/late', 'doctors' round delayed', 'no room available', 'midwife not available', 'doctor not available'. The most common reason (65%) for delay was that the doctors' round was delayed. This is obviously unavoidable at times. However, by asking mothers to ring before setting out to the hospital, delays for induction because there are no rooms available have been eliminated.

Clearly it is not possible to eliminate all delays on a labour suite, but this demonstrates that by introducing simple changes, it is possible to reduce the number of mothers who wait long periods of time to be induced.

Care of Mothers who have a Stillbirth or Fetal Loss

Most labours have a happy outcome, but sadly, some do

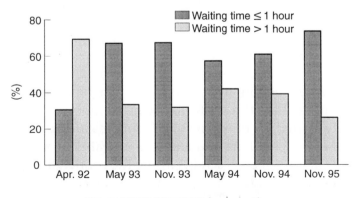

Figure 8.5 Waiting times for induction.

not. Midwifery practice has moved on a long way since the days when babies who were stillborn were taken away from their mothers without their mothers being given the chance to see or hold them. Although care had improved, the Labour Suite Standard Setting Group felt there was a need to have better guidelines about what investigations needed to be done in what circumstances, practical information about how samples should be taken, research findings about fetal loss and information about supporting grieving parents. The group set a standard: 'Every midwife will be aware of the procedure for managing and supporting a mother who has had a stillbirth or pregnancy loss, and will have access to support for her/himself if necessary.' To implement the standard, a manual of information for staff covering subjects such as support of mothers, how to carry out tests, and research literature was produced. It is easily accessible on the labour suite.

The Labour Suite Standard Setting Group also developed guidelines summarizing the main things to be done, people to inform, and documentation to complete according to whether the mother has a stillbirth, miscarriage or termination of pregnancy. The chart is a tick list and is completed for every mother who has a fetal loss or stillbirth. It is then filed in the back of the casenotes as part of the documentation and as a record of the tests that have been carried out so that investigations are not repeated, as well as evidence that appropriate people have been informed.

As part of the standard, a memento book was developed by a midwife at the Nottingham City Hospital Maternity Unit. The book is given to all mothers who have had a stillbirth or miscarriage as a way of preserving mementos of their baby. It is a small book with A6 plastic pockets. The opening pages consist of information about the grieving process, contact numbers and a poem. The remaining pages consist of decorated cards with space for parents to place keepsakes of their baby, for example a lock of hair, the baby's name band, photographs and footprints. They are also available in Asian languages. Parents appreciate the memento book and we have received much positive verbal and written feedback about this innovation.

Postnatal care

Privacy

An early standard set by the Ward Standard Setting Group before *The Patient's Charter* (Department of Health, 1991) was produced on the subject of privacy. Staff, be they midwifery, medical or domestic, had always been somewhat casual about wandering into rooms or behind curtains without checking whether it was appropriate to do so. The standard was set that 'every woman is offered privacy whilst on the ward.' Midwifery staff were asked to ensure that domestic and medical staff respected mothers' privacy and mothers were told on admission to the ward that they could draw the curtains around the bed if they wished or put up the 'do not disturb' notice at the door if in a side ward.

The standard was monitored by asking mothers the following three questions on the day of discharge: 'Did you want privacy whilst on the ward?' 'Did you feel you were offered privacy?' and 'Did you feel able to obtain privacy if you wanted it?' *Figure 8.6* shows the results of the audits.

It is interesting to note the low figures for the question 'Did you want privacy whilst on the ward?' Only about half the mothers said they did. This was a consistent finding. Mothers did not seem to perceive a need for privacy whilst on the ward although they clearly felt that they were offered it and could obtain it if needed. The audit results show an improvement in mothers feeling able to

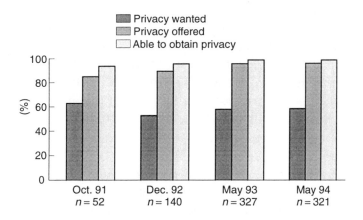

Figure 8.6 *Results of audits on privacy.*

obtain and being offered privacy over a period of four years. This standard has been amended to apply to all areas of the maternity unit.

Information about Vitamin K

Since the 1950s it has been common practice to give newborn babies vitamin K to prevent the occurrence of haemorrhagic disease of the newborn, though this practice has often been the subject of debate (Handel and Tripp, 1991). An important part of the midwife's role is to inform mothers about the reason for giving vitamin K and to obtain informed consent. In our unit, however, it had been reported that at times mothers were not getting an explanation, especially at night, and that sometimes nursing auxiliaries were giving the explanation. The Standard Setting Group looking at the care of babies felt that these practices were unacceptable. A standard was therefore set stating that 'All babies will be offered vitamin K with the informed consent of the mother or father.' Midwives were reminded of the need to give an explanation and to obtain verbal consent from every mother before giving vitamin K.

The standard was audited by asking mothers on the day of discharge 'Did your baby have vitamin K drops?' 'Did you understand why your baby had vitamin K drops?' It was decided to word the second question in the past tense to test whether mothers felt that they had been given an understandable explanation at the time of administration as it did not seem fair to expect mothers to remember an explanation that may have been given several days before.

The results of the audits were considered to be fairly satisfactory, but it was felt that mothers' understanding of the use of vitamin K could be better, particularly as at the time research had been published that appeared to link the administration of intramuscular vitamin K with childhood cancers (Golding *et al.*, 1992). As a consequence, an information sheet was produced to be given to all mothers by the midwife to supplement the verbal explanation. This has now been laminated and is placed at every bedside. The results of the audits are shown in *Figure 8.7*.

The information sheet was introduced between the third and fourth audit and it is interesting to note the improvement in the percentage of mothers who said they understood the explanation. 92.5% said they had received the information sheet.

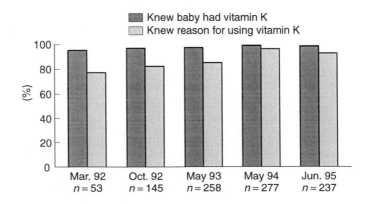

Figure 8.7 Mothers' understanding of the use of vitamin K.

Information about Cot Death

In 1991, the Department of Health (1991b) issued guide-lines about reducing the risk of cot death, producing a leaflet which summarized four ways to reduce the risks as placing babies on their backs to sleep, not overheating babies, not exposing babies to cigarette smoke, and informing the doctor if a baby is unwell.

Midwives are key health professionals in their role of advising and giving information and support to new mothers and it was felt that this was a vitally important area. A standard was therefore set that stated that 'all mothers will be aware of the measures to be taken to reduce the risk of cot death, in the light of recent research.'

To implement the standard, education sessions were arranged for all staff, including nursing auxiliaries, about the latest guidelines. Every mother was to be given a copy of the Department of Health leaflet *Reduce the Risk of Cot Death* before she went home in addition to verbal advice.

An attractive nursery thermometer was also made available along with a leaflet produced by the Foundation for the Study of Infant Deaths (FSID) called *Reducing the Risk of Cot Death* (FSID, 1992). These are sold to mothers on the wards and through parentcraft for a small sum and are another way of helping mothers to reduce the risk of cot death by highlighting the impor-tance of not overheating babies.

To audit the standard, we asked mothers whether they knew how to reduce the risk of cot death and whether they received a copy of the Department of Health leaflet. The results of several audits can be seen in *Figure 8.8*. The lower percentage of mothers receiving the leaflet in the second was thought to result from ask-ing some mothers whether they had received the leaflet before they had been given it at discharge. It was subse-quently decided to give the leaflet to mothers on the first day after delivery.

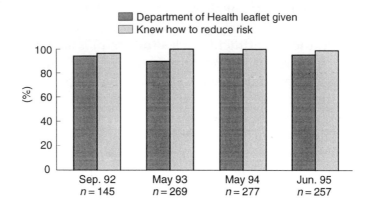

Figure 8.8 *Results of audits on informing mothers how to reduce the risk of cot death.*

Although midwives cannot claim all the credit for mothers knowing how to reduce the risk of cot death it is satisfying to be able to demonstrate that mothers are at least leaving hospital with this knowledge. An account of this initiative has been published (Buckley, 1993).

Cot death and smoking. Linked in with this standard, and also to complement the standard on smoking set by the Antenatal Clinic Standard Setting Group, a short questionnaire was designed and produced in the form of a sticker (*Figure 8.9*), which is attached onto the postnatal discharge page in the casenotes. Mothers are asked whether they or their partner smokes and if so, how many cigarettes did they smoke the day before delivery. These data are subsequently entered onto a computer. If the mother or father smokes, the question is asked 'How do you think smoking might affect your baby?' The prompts remind the midwife about the ways in which babies can be affected by cigarette smoke so that the information can be given to the mother. The mother is then asked how she is going to provide a 'smoke-free zone' for her baby. Again, there are prompts for the midwife to make suggestions. Use of the questionnaire has been audited and it was found that 88% of mothers had been advised about the effects of smoking

POSTNATAL QUESTIONNAIRE ON SMOKING

PLEASE ASK ALL MOTHERS THE FOLLOWING QUESTIONS:
1. DO YOU, OR DOES YOUR PARTNER SMOKE?   YES/NO

IF NO, DISCUSS IMPORTANCE OF NOT EXPOSING BABY TO <u>ANY</u> SMOKY ENVIRONMENT.
                                                     ADVICE GIVEN?   YES/NO
IF YES, ASK:
2. HOW MANY CIGARETTES DID YOU SMOKE THE DAY BEFORE YOU DELIVERED?
.... DAY   PARTNER? .... DAY

3. HOW DO YOU THINK SMOKING MIGHT AFFECT YOUR BABY? (SMOKING INCREASES THE
RISK OF COT DEATH 2–5 FOLD, ASTHMA, CHEST INFECTIONS AND GLUE EAR)
                                                     ADVICE GIVEN?   YES/NO

4. HOW ARE YOU GOING TO PROVIDE A 'SMOKE-FREE ZONE' FOR YOUR BABY?
(SUGGESTIONS: GIVE UP SMOKING; SMOKE OUTSIDE AND ASK OTHERS TO; DON'T SMOKE IN
THE SAME ROOM AS THE BABY; SMOKE BY OPEN WINDOW)
                                                     ADVICE GIVEN?   YES/NO

SIGNATURE ....   DATE ....

© Nottingham City Hospital Maternity Unit, 1994, 1996

Figure 8.9 *Postnatal questionnaire on smoking.*

and 82% had been asked and advised about providing a 'smoke-free zone' for the baby.

Other Postnatal Standards

Other standards set by the Ward and Care of Babies Standard Setting Groups concern orientating mothers to the ward (a ward information leaflet was produced) and supporting mothers who breastfeed, and those mothers who want to help with tube feeding their babies (a leaflet was produced). Giving information about Guthrie tests, postnatal exercises and making up bottle feeds are the subjects of other standards.

Unit standards

As many aspects of care in individual areas were covered, the way ahead seemed to be to broaden the

approach to standard setting. After several years of setting standards in specific areas, it was decided to disband the Standard Setting Groups and take a fresh look
at what needed to be done and what staff felt were the
important issues. All Nottingham City Hospital
Maternity Unit staff were given the opportunity to suggest topics for consideration and to be involved in standard setting groups. Below are some of the broader
issues addressed in standard setting groups.

Interpreting Cardiotocographs (CTGs)

Although CTGs have been part of obstetric and midwifery care since the 1960s, interpretation has never been
straightforward and they have at times seemed more of a
hindrance than a help to good obstetric and midwifery
care. In a small proportion of babies abnormal CTGs have
been found to be an indication of birth asphyxia, which
may lead to significant fetal morbidity or mortality (Gibb
and Arulkumaran, 1992; Ingemarrson *et al.*, 1993). CTGs
are often used in evidence in litigation. The *Confidential
Enquiry into Stillbirths and Deaths in Infancy* (CESDI) in its
Annual Reports in 1993 and 1994 (Department of Health,
1995, 1996) found that a significant number of deaths
were at least contributed to by failure to interpret and act
on abnormal CTGs. Problems sometimes arose because
abnormalities were not recognized or because there were
no clear guidelines or agreement on what the trace
meant. They recommended training in interpretation and
clear guidelines on when to act.

Midwives and doctors in working at Nottingham
City Hospital Maternity Unit had the same concerns. A
group of midwives and obstetricians was formed to
look at the interpretation of CTGs. It is an enormous
subject and knowing where to start was difficult. The
group looked at the issues surrounding interpretation:
definitions, classification, assessment, accountability,

documentation and education. These were illustrated in a flow chart, which was split into the two main areas: antepartum CTGs and intrapartum CTGs. A standard was set stating that 'all midwives and obstetric staff will be able to recognize normal and abnormal cardiotocographs (CTGs) and take appropriate clinical action in accordance with the Unit policy'.

The subject of antepartum CTGs was looked at first and a variety of references were used including several recent books on the subject and the recommendations of the Fédération Internationale de Gynécologie et Obstétrique (FIGO, 1987).

Draft guidelines were distributed to wards, departments, midwives and obstetricians for comment. Guidelines were produced for the interpretation of antepartum CTGs, intrapartum CTGs 1st stage and intrapartum CTGs 2nd stage. They contain definitions, classifications and principles for assessment and action. They also address documentation and storage of CTGs. All staff are expected to follow the protocol. They are in laminated form on all wards and in all labour suite rooms. Handy 'credit card' size copies of the guidelines were produced for staff to buy. A computer-assisted learning package is used for staff for updating midwives and doctors and the induction of new staff. The standard has been audited.

Postnatal Haemoglobins

Postnatal anaemia is a common problem in the puerperium. It is defined as a haemaglobin (Hb) concentration of less than 10 g/dl (World Health Organization, 1972) and affects 20–40% of women (Richter *et al.*, 1995). Postpartum anaemia is associated with maternal fatigue, dizziness, breathlessness and the 'blues' (Paterson *et al.*, 1994; Meyer *et al.*, 1995).

It was decided to audit postnatal Hb concentrations

over one year using the discharge data input on the computer, and it was found that 22.2% mothers had a Hb of less than 10 g/dl and 9.2% had a Hb concentration less than or equal to 9 g/dl. The method of delivery had the greatest effect on the postnatal Hb: 26% of mothers having instrumental deliveries had a low Hb compared with 4.6% of mothers having normal deliveries. The results were presented at the Maternal Morbidity and Perinatal Mortality Meetings and the results were discussed.

It was decided to aim to halve the number of low postnatal Hb concentrations. Guidelines were formulated as a result of suggestions from midwifery and obstetric staff. These were mainly simple suggestions, for example how to reduce blood loss at delivery by keeping the bladder empty, prompt perineal suturing, and prompt administration of Syntometrine. Three lists of guidelines were produced aimed at midwives, doctors carrying out instrumental deliveries and surgeons carrying out caesarian sections.

The guidelines and results in graph form are displayed in the labour suite, the wards, and theatre. Monthly results are presented at the Perinatal Mortality Meeting. Displaying results increases awareness of the issues. *Figure 8.10* and *8.11* show the monthly results overall and for normal delivery.

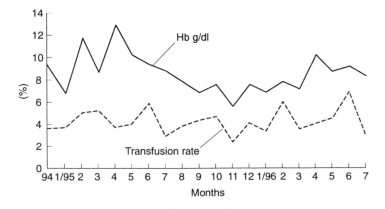

Figure 8.10 Postnatal haemoglobin (Hb) concentrations and transfusion rates

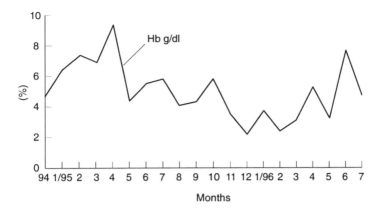

Figure 8.11 *Percentage of women with a normal delivery and a low postnatal haemoglobin (Hb) concentration.*

The initial aim of reducing the number of low postnatal Hb concentrations by 50% over the period of one year has been found to be too ambitious. However, the overall aim remains the same. In the year since the initiative was started there has been a 16% reduction in the number of low Hb concentrations. Minimizing blood loss at delivery is good midwifery and obstetric practice, reduces maternal morbidity, and makes more efficient use of resources.

Security

Ever since the abduction of Abbie Humphreys from Queen's Medical Centre, Nottingham in 1993, the security of babies has been a concern of maternity units all over the UK. We installed an electronic tagging system, but had a lot of 'false alarms'. A standard was set with the aim of reducing the false alarms. An audit was carried out of when and why the false alarms took place. As a result we changed the procedure of when tags were removed from babies and what was done with them with a resulting fall in the number of false alarms. A laminated leaflet was produced for mothers to read and is by every bed on the wards.

Ethnic Issues

The Patient's Charter Standard number 1 (Department of Health, 1991b) states that patients should be given 'respect for privacy, dignity and religious and cultural beliefs.' A group was therefore set up to look at these issues in Nottingham City Hospital Maternity Unit. The Unit already had an interpreter who was available to translate for Asian mothers, leaflets about pregnancy in Asian languages, and the Department of Health (1991b) leaflet *Reduce the Risk of Cot Death* in nine languages. In addition, the ward information leaflet, the vitamin K information leaflet, the Bacille Calmette–Guérin (BCG) leaflet and audio cassettes containing the same information were produced in Asian languages.

Visitors

The Labour Suite Standard Setting Group reported an apparent increase in visitor incidents. Staff were asked to document any incidents in a book over a period of 16 months. The incidents recorded were rudeness, verbal abuse, uncooperation and invasion of privacy. An account of this initiative has been published (Buckley, 1995). As a result guidelines were developed for visitors and staff were encouraged to be firm with visitors, not to tolerate abuse and to report serious incidents to security. Incident forms are now completed for serious problems. A hospital group has been started to look at the issues, partly as a result of the problems highlighted in the Maternity Unit.

Problems with visitors appears to be a relatively recent phenomenon, but one which is, in general, being taken more seriously.

Back Care

Setting standards and quality initiatives need not necessarily be always about patient care. Back problems are a common and serious cause of morbidity in midwives (Royal College of Midwives, 1993). A standard was therefore set aimed at raising awareness of what maternity staff could do to reduce the risk of back injury. Three posters were produced: *Helping to Prevent Back Problems* gives general guidelines such as regular exercise and, wearing non-slip shoes; *General Principles of Lifting* gives advice such as get help if you need it, keep your spine in a natural line, kneel or crouch rather than stoop; and *Guidelines When Lifting Patients* advises lifting with a person of similar build, eliminating hazards if possible, and using an appropriate handling method. These are displayed on the wards and labour suite.

Care Cards

The 'Care Card' scheme at Nottingham City Hospital Maternity Unit was started in 1991 at the suggestion of two ultrasonographers who had been to a study day where the scheme had been discussed at another hospital. At booking, mothers who have experienced a personal tragedy which may cause anxiety or sadness in the pregnancy (often a stillbirth or neonatal loss) are identified by the midwife. The mother is told about the scheme whereby her casenotes and cooperation card can be identified by a silver star (if she wishes), and she is offered a 'Care Card' which she shows at antenatal visits. The star on the casenotes or cooperation card alert staff so that mothers can be treated with extra sensitivity.

The system was audited by a computer program, which automatically produced a questionnaire along with the discharge letter which the midwife used to ask the mothers questions about how useful they found the card. Eighty percent of mothers found it useful and 89% found that staff were sympathetic. There was a lack of knowledge about the purpose of the card among medical staff, particularly registrars and senior house officers. A poster was therefore produced summarizing the scheme and is displayed in the doctors' room on the labour suite.

Conclusions

The standards and quality initiatives discussed in this chapter demonstrate some of the work carried out at Nottingham City Hospital Maternity Unit. Some ideas have worked better than others. Some standards have proved difficult to audit and have gone by the wayside. However, the successes outnumber the failures and the unit has demonstrated that it is possible to set standards, evaluate care and make changes improve care.

Perhaps the most important point is that standards should relate to important issues, either subjects felt to be a particular problem or a specific professional or clinical matter, and be related if possible, to other national or local standards or government targets. Standard setting is time consuming and expensive in terms of resources. The time and effort should be used effectively and efficiently to address those matters that affect outcomes and can significantly improve care. Just as important is that standards are monitored regularly in order to demonstrate that the improvement is actually taking place.

Key points

- Standards should be set on important issues, relating them where possible to existing local or national standards.

- All standards should be monitored, but timing should be flexible.

- Some standards will work better than others.

References

Bennett V and Brown L (1989) *Myles Textbook for Midwives*, 11th Edition. Churchill Livingstone: London. p. 205.

Bobak I and Jensen M (1989) *Maternity and Gynaecologic Care*. Mosby: St, Louis. p. 441.

Buckley ER (1991a) Why do we have to wait so long? *Midwives Chronicle* **104** (1242): 196–199.

Buckley ER (1991b) *Mostly waiting*. Midwifery Information and Resource Service (MIDIRS) **1**(4): 413–416.

Buckley ER (1993) Reducing the risk. *Nursing Times* October 23rd: 28–30.

Buckley ER (1995) How much of a problem are visitors on labour suite? *British Journal of Midwifery* **3** (3): 138–170.

Department of Health (1991a) *The Patient's Charter*. HMSO: London.

Department of Health (1991b) *Reduce the Risk of Cot Death*. HMSO: London.

Department of Health (1992) *Health of the Nation*. HMSO: London. p. 18.

Department of Health (1995) *Confidential Enquiry into Stillbirths and Deaths in Infancy: Annual Report from 1 January–31 December 1993*. HMSO: London.

Department of Health (1996) *Confidential Enquiry into Stillbirths and Deaths in Infancy: Annual Report from 1 January–31 December 1994*. HMSO: London.

Fédération Internationale de Gynécologie et d'Obstétrique (1987) Guidelines for the use of fetal monitoring. *International Journal of Gynaecology and Obstetrics* **25**: 159–167.

Foundation for the Study of Infant Deaths (1992) *Reducing The Risk of Cot Death*. FSID: London.

Gibb D and Arulkumaran S (1992) *Fetal Monitoring in Practice*. Butterworth Heinemann: Oxford. p. 146.

Golding J, Greenwood R and Mott M (1992) Childhood cancer, intramuscular vitamin K, and pethidine given during labour. *British Medical Journal* **305**: 341–346.

Handel J and Tripp J (1991) Vitamin K prophylaxis against haemorrhagic disease of the newborn in the United Kingdom. *British Medical Journal* **303**: 1109.

Howie P (1995) The physiology of the puerperium and lactation. In: Chamberlain G (ed.) *Turnbull's Obstetrics*, 2nd edn. Churchill Livingstone: London. p. 756.

Ingemarrson I, Ingemarrson E and Spencer J (1993) *Fetal Heart Monitoring*. Oxford University Press: Oxford. pp. 260, 291.

Meyer J Eichhorn K, Vetter K, *et al.* (1995) Does recombinant erythropoietin not only treat anaemia but reduce postpartum (emotional) distress as well? *Journal of Perinatal Medicine* **23**: 99–109.

Paterson J, Davis J and Gregory M *et al.* (1994) A study on the effects of low haemoglobin on postnatal women. *Midwifery* **10** (2): 77–86.

Prochaska J and DiClemente C (1983) Stages and processes of self-change of smoking toward an integrative model of change. *Journal of Consulting and Clinical Psychology* **51**: 390–395.

Richter C, Huch A and Huch R (1995) Erythropoiesis in the postpartum period. *Journal of Perinatal Medicine* **23**: 51–59.

Royal College of Midwives (1993) *Handbook for Health and Safety Representatives.* Royal College of Midwives: London. p. 5.

Silargy C, Lancaster T, Fowler G and Spiers I (1996) *Effectiveness of Training Health Professionals to Provide Smoking Cessation Interventions: Systematic Review of Randomised Controlled Trials.* Cochrane Library Issue 2.

Sleep J, Roberts J and Chalmers I (1989) *Care During the Second Stage of Labour. Effective Care in Pregnancy.* Oxford University Press: Oxford. p. 1136.

Smith D, Slack R and Marteau T (1994) Lack of knowledge in health professionals: a barrier to providing information for parents? *Quality in Health Care* **3**: 75–78.

Whent H (1994) *Smoking and Pregnancy. Guidance for Purchasers and Providers.* Health Education Authority: London. pp. 2–3.

World Health Organization (1972) *Nutritional Anaemias.* Technical Report Series 503.

Section 5 The Future of Quality

9 Quality in Midwifery – Where Now?

'How can we know where we are going if we do not know where we are?' (Margaret Auld, Royal College of Midwives' conference 1980).

'In the end, quality must be seen whole, not in fragmented parts' (Maxwell, 1984).

Quality and audit in the health professions seemed to come out of nowhere in the 1980s. The concept has in a short space of time infiltrated policies, procedures, contracts, education and literature. But, in a few years' time, will it disappear as quickly as it arose? It has been suggested that audit may have run out of steam (Thomson and Barton, 1994), and it has even been questioned whether audit and quality issues are valid at all.

Bulstrode *et al.* (1993) concluded that '...the future of audit must be questionable.'

What is the future for quality, and more specifically for quality in midwifery? Is it a passing phase or is it here to stay?

Quality is here to stay

Quality issues have been around since the beginning of time. People have always measured their expectations and standards against reality. Only relatively recently have they been formalized into 'quality and audit issues'.

Although giving quality care has always been important to midwives, again, it is only relatively recently that midwives have looked objectively at their practice and started to evaluate it. Until then, changes were generally driven by obstetricians, lay bodies and government, and occasionally research. Over the last few years midwives have started to take the initiative and to look at their practice, demonstrating that they are giving quality, research-based care and producing good outcomes.

Quality is here to stay for three main reasons: professionally it is of the utmost importance that midwives demonstrate to themselves and others, particularly those they care for, that their care is competent and effective; the government requires that health professionals constantly evaluate and improve their practice; and quality clauses are becoming more common in contracts.

Quality issues are here to stay, and midwives need to be at the centre of initiatives aimed at improving the quality of care for mothers and babies.

All Midwives Should be Involved in Audit and Quality Issues

Audit and quality issues are not just for the specialist or

the enthusiast. They are for everybody. Using a simple but flexible method of setting and implementing standards which involves everyone is the way forward. This ethos of quality and audit being everybody's business should be an integral part of midwife education and a major thread running through post-registration education.

Quality is a process, not an event

The process of implementing quality never stands still. It is a dynamic process, not a one-off event. As new research emerges and professional and government recommendations are produced, midwives need to look at the totality of care, not just one small part, taking into account the broader as well as the narrower issues of midwifery care.

Autonomy and standards

Midwives have a great deal of autonomy and are accountable for their own practice (United Kingdom Central Council for Nursing, Midwifery and Health Visiting, 1994). They have always been proud of their independent practitioner status. However, they need to be careful that this autonomy does not lure them away from the safety of giving research-based care, based on standards produced by consensus. Margaret Auld, in a paper given at the Royal College of Midwives' Annual Professional Day in 1979, said that 'midwives have not attempted to evaluate with any degree of accuracy or certainty the care given, nor have we established a code of good practice' (Auld, 1980).

It is a matter of concern that midwives and midwifery have so far failed in any large part to involve themselves in setting standards (Dawson, 1993). Indeed it may be

that midwives have become fixated about their independent status and their need to protect it. This may have
hindered them from looking further than the one to one
individualized care of mother and baby to the broader
professional issues of consensus standards, which both
nursing and medicine have embraced.

Midwifery care, and in particular the professional
progress of the last few years, must to be safeguarded by
research-based practice. Things have progressed from
the days when Cochrane (1979) stated that 'it is in
obstetrics and gynaecology in which clinical practice is
least likely to be supported by clinical evidence.'
However, not all practice is yet based on research findings and it is important that midwives in their zeal to
give individualized care do not stray from evidence-
based guidelines.

Top-down or bottom-up?

There are many approaches to quality and although
these systems have been applied to health care, there is
little in the literature to suggest which is the most successful approach in midwifery. Is the future of quality in
midwifery in top-down quality systems like *Total Quality
Management* (TQM) or in bottom-up quality improvement such as the Royal College of Nursing's DySSSY
system or standard setting as described in this book?

TQM is an organization-wide approach based on
broad objectives, which are designed to affect every part
of the organization at all levels. It requires huge
resources in terms of training and mobilizing all staff.
Although top-down systems can no doubt work in midwifery and maternity services, bottom-up approaches
are easier to get going and changes can be made and
problems tackled relatively quickly. It has been shown
that a standard setting approach, as described in this

book, can be successful in implementing change. It may be that bottom-up approaches are a necessary forerunner of an organization-wide approach like TQM.

The bottom-up approach appears to be the way ahead in the government's thinking when it states that 'audit should be clinically led', 'focused on the patient', 'within a culture of constant evaluation of clinical effectiveness focusing on patient outcomes', but also linked into existing quality and audit initiatives (Department of Health, 1994).

It is clear that quality initiatives and standards need to be grounded 'on the shop floor'. As the current emphasis is on multiprofessional audit and quality, auditing outcomes and each taking responsibility for his/her own practice, it is likely that the most effective quality improvement initiatives are those initiated at or near the level of the shop floor. The control of projects, changes and evaluation of outcomes should be kept firmly in clinician's hands.

Multidisciplinary or undisciplinary?

There has been a move towards multidisciplinary audit in recent years. The term 'medical audit' is increasingly being replaced by 'clinical audit' as it is recognized that audit is not solely a medical activity, but one that involves all the clinicians responsible for a given service. The Department of Health recognized that there is a place for both uniprofessional and multiprofessional audit in its document *Clinical Audit* (1993). Some subjects do not involve other disciplines, for example, breast-feeding, ward orientation, while other topics of interest or identified issues, for example interpretation of cardiotocographs, will involve other disciplines. A flexible approach is needed. Involving other disciplines for standards that do not involve them is a waste of time and resources.

Quality coordinators

'Clinical audit must remain clinically led' (Department of Health, 1993). 'A leader should be identified within each healthcare team to motivate and cascade change within the team' (Department of Health, 1994).

If quality in midwifery is to be 'clinically led', it needs management support input and it needs to be co-ordinated. As discussed in Chapter 4, initiating quality and audit takes time and resources and can not be carried out by a midwife with a full clinical workload. The way ahead is to appoint a midwife to coordinate quality and audit and to make this a recognized grade and career step that stays firmly based within the maternity unit or health centre.

Building on what is already there

Introducing quality does not mean reinventing the wheel. It builds on the good things which are already there, using the existing structures and processes effectively eliminating obsolete or ineffective practices, targeting information more accurately. It also integrates with other quality and audit activities (Department of Health, 1994).

Computerization, ownership and access

Love them or loathe them, computers are here to stay. Most maternity units enter clinical data onto some sort of computer system, and it is likely that this will be the trend for maternity units in the future. As computer systems become widespread, they will become integrated with other services. Systems such as Hospital Information Systems (HISS) where all departments in the hospital and general practices are on one system and able to access and update data will become commonplace. The potential for using these systems for audit projects will be tremendous.

Computerization has advantages and a disadvantages. Being able to access information, avoiding duplication and improving communication are a few of the advantages. However, it is ironic that those advantages can turn into the disadvantages when computers do not work properly, creating extra work, increasing stress if the systems are slow, and increasing the risk to mothers if information is not accessible because of breakdown. Training issues should not be underestimated. There is also the danger that the data will not be easily accessible to ordinary clinicians, but only to managers and information technology departments (Crombie and Davies, 1991). It is important that clinicians keep their 'finger on the pulse' and when new systems are being considered that they take an active part, make the requirement that data relevant to auditing practice are collected, and are themselves able to access data easily, preferably directly, so that they can use them for their own practice.

There is also the issue of ownership to consider. It is vital that clinicians remain the guardians of clinical data and that it is not hijacked by general managers and administrators.

Publication

Until recently it was hard to find any specific literature or statements about quality and audit issues in midwifery. Medicine, nursing and the other therapies are well ahead of midwifery in this respect. The future of quality in midwifery depends to a large extent on midwives not only measuring, evaluating and improving their service and practice in collaboration with other health professionals as appropriate, but in disseminating their findings in midwifery and medical journals so that others can benefit.

Conclusion

'Outcomes, by and large, remain the ultimate validation of the effectiveness and quality of medical care' (Donabedian, 1966). The principle applies just as much to midwifery care. The future of quality in midwifery does not lie merely in the direction of 'woman-centred care'. More than ever, midwives need to ensure that the care they give is based on evidence-based consensus standards. More than that, midwives need to evaluate their practice, implementing change on the basis of the findings and disseminating their work. Then they really will be able to claim that they are 'delivering quality'.

Key points

- Quality issues are here to stay.

- Quality is a process not an event.

- Bottom-up approaches are those most likely to work in midwifery.

- Quality coordinators should be appointed in every maternity unit and community service.

- Midwifery practice should be based on evidence-based consensus standards.

- Midwives should be able to access data for audit purposes.

- Quality initiatives and changes based on the implementation of audit results should be disseminated widely in journals and at conferences.

- Quality is for everybody.

References

Auld M (1980) Midwifery standards. *Midwives' Chronicle and Nursing Notes* January 1980: 5–11.

Bulstrode C, Carr A, Pynsent P and Wildner M (1993) Audit: Will it work? Quoted in: Frostick P, Radford PJ, Wallace WA (eds) *Medical Audit Rationale and Practicalities.* Cambridge University Press: Cambridge. p. 413.

Cochrane A (1979) 1931–1971: A critical review with particular reference to the medical profession. In: *Medicine for the Year 2000.* Office of Health Economics: London. pp. 2–11.

Crombie I and Davies T (1991) Computers in audit: servants or sirens? *British Medical Journal* 303: 403–404.

Dawson J (1993) The role of quality assurance in future midwifery practice. *Journal of Advanced Nursing* 18: 1251–1258.

Department of Health (1993) *Clinical Audit. Meeting and Improving Standards in Health Care.* HMSO: London. p. 13.

Department of Health (1994) *The Evolution of Clinical Audit.* HMSO: London. p. 15.

Donabedian A (1966) *Evaluating the Quality of Medical Care.* Millbank Memorial Fund Quarterly 44: 166–203.

Maxwell R (1984) Quality assessment in health. *British Medical Journal* 288: 1470–1472.

Royal College of Nursing (1990) *Quality Patient Care: An Introduction to the RCN Dynamic Standard Setting System (DySSSy).* Scutari Press: London.

Thomson R and Barton A (1994) Is audit running out of steam? *Quality in Health Care* 3: 225–229.

United Kingdom Central Council for Nursing, Midwifery and Health Visiting (1994) *The Midwife's Code of Practice.* UKCC: London. p. 3.

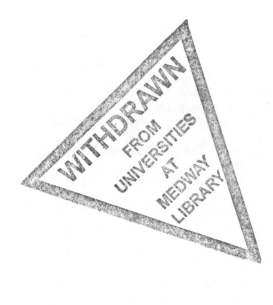

Index